BEAST MODE
— FOR THE —
MODERN MAN

HOW TO GROW INSIDE AND OUTSIDE THE GYM

LEVEL UP
CO. PRESS

First edition

ISBN: 978-1-923014-49-7

"To our families and partners, thank you for being our pillars of support and strength as we embarked on this journey. To the beautiful team of people, we have in our lives constantly pushing us to unleash our inner beasts, this book is for you….!"

- The Level Up Co Press Beasts

CONTENTS

AUTHOR'S REFLECTIONS: SHARING THE VISION

In a world where societal expectations often define what it means to be a man, we felt compelled to challenge the status quo. As men ourselves, we recognized the pressing need for a fresh perspective, one that celebrates personal growth, resilience, and a holistic approach to well-being. This realization led us to embark on a journey to write "Beast Mode for the Modern Man: How to Grow Inside and Outside the Gym."

As we explored the struggles faced by men today, we couldn't ignore the alarming trends we witnessed. Men were increasingly burdened by sleep deprivation, stress, burnout, and a lack of exercise and proper nutrition. Furthermore, a disheartening lack of financial literacy seemed to pervade our gender. It became clear that a paradigm shift was essential, empowering men to break free from these limitations and reclaim their power.

This book is not a mere collection of theories or idealistic dreams. Instead, it draws from our own personal experiences, successes, and failures. We have implemented the strategies and techniques outlined in these pages, witnessing firsthand their transformative impact personally and for our clients. We offer them not as mere suggestions, but as battle-tested tools for change.

Our aim is simple: to encourage men to develop a beast mode mentality, a powerful mindset and attitude that empowers them to take control and take action. By addressing the physical, mental, and financial aspects of their lives, we seek to guide men towards a state of optimal well-being and fulfilment. "Beast Mode for the Modern Man" is more than a self-help book; it's a call to action. We challenge the myths that confine masculinity and encourage men to embrace their authentic selves. Within these chapters, you will find real world solutions, practical strategies, and actionable advice that will propel you towards a life of vitality and purpose.

ABOUT THE AUTHORS

Level Up Co. Press is an international publishing company that was established by a team of experts who are passionate about sharing their knowledge and experiences with others. The company's board of experts boasts diverse professional backgrounds that encompass financial services, money management, business operations, sales and marketing, health, fitness and nutrition, and relationships.

Their collective knowledge is utilized to provide practical advice and expertise to men, women, and teenagers, with the ultimate goal of helping individuals improve their lives and unleash their inner beasts!

These modern men come with real results and believe in providing high-quality content that is both informative and engaging, with books that cover a range of topics to empower individuals to make positive changes and achieve their goals.

Level Up Co Press is always looking to improve and expand its offerings, inviting readers to join them on a journey of discovery, growth, and transformation.

HERE'S WHAT SOME OF THEIR CLIENTS HAVE TO SAY

"I have had the pleasure of working with an incredible financial professional for several years now, and their expertise has helped me tremendously in managing my personal wealth. Their guidance and strategies have allowed me to achieve financial goals that I never thought were possible. I was thrilled to learn that they have recently contributed to publishing a book series, which is a testament to their vast knowledge and experience in this field. Their book is a must-read for anyone who wants to take control of their finances and build a secure financial future."

Financially back on Track

"I have been working with my personal trainer for years now, and I can confidently say that he is one of the best in the business. He understands that weight loss is not just about exercise, but also about nutrition, and he helped me get my diet on track before introducing me to a workout regime that was perfect for my needs. With his guidance and support, I was able to drop a significant amount of body fat percentage and pack on a reasonable amount of muscle mass over the past 12 months. I was unhappy and not confident at all in myself. I am so grateful for his expertise, dedication, and encouragement throughout this journey, and I would recommend him to anyone who is serious about getting fit and healthy."

Feeling Fit and Healthy

"I have had the pleasure of working with my mentor for several years now, and I can say without a doubt that he has had a profound impact on both my personal and professional growth. As a high flying corporate responsible for managing over 100 staff, I have learned from him the importance of leading with integrity and prioritizing the needs, feelings, and thoughts of those around me. Through his guidance and support, I have been able to scale up my business to great success by becoming the best manager I can be.

My mentor and I regularly engage in blue sky think tanks, where we envision the future growth of the business and work on developing a growth mindset that keeps me accountable to my goals and dreams. He has helped me understand the value of building relationships with those around me, and I am forever grateful for the wisdom he has imparted.

I am excited to learn that he has collaborated with other professionals on a book, and I look forward to reading it. I can wholeheartedly recommend him to anyone who is seeking to grow personally or professionally."

Grateful for your Wisdom

The information contained within this book is general in nature and has not taken your personal circumstances into consideration. It is provided for informational purposes only, and the strategies outlined may not be suitable for everyone. Therefore, we strongly recommend seeking professional advice before entering into any financial, nutritional, physical exercise programs or taking on any relationship advice. The strategies within this book have purely been strategies used and implemented in the lives of the Authors and have provided real-life results for them as individuals. However, the authors do not guarantee any specific outcomes or results, and readers should use their discretion when implementing any of the strategies discussed in this book.

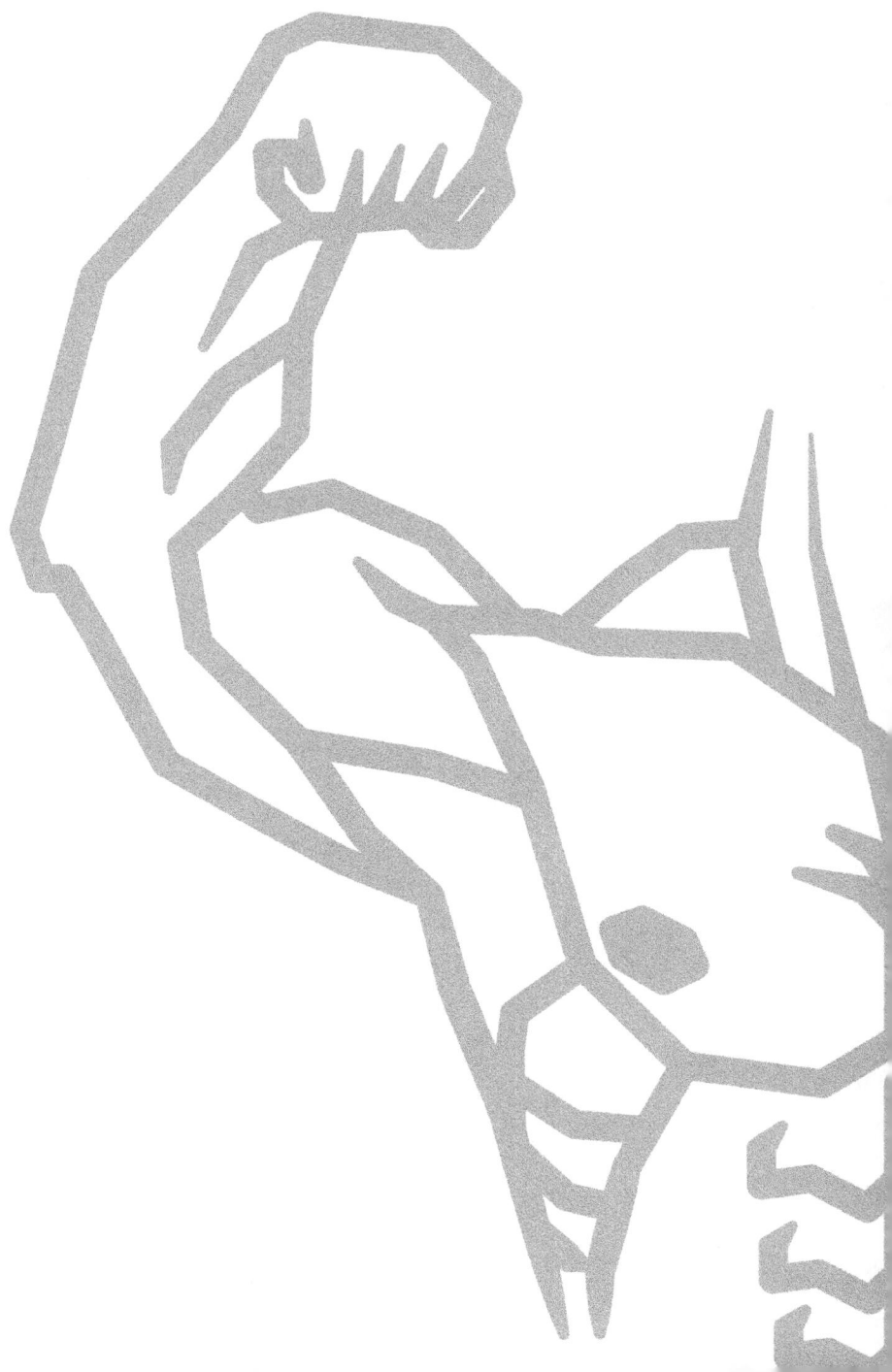

INTRODUCTION

From childhood, we have repeatedly heard the phrase, "be a man," haven't we? This statement is flawed, and it burdens men with unrealistic expectations and harms their self-respect. Men get the message that they lack certain masculine characteristics. Our society tries to paint a distinct picture of what men "should" and "shouldn't" do; however, these paradigms need to change.

In our society, being sensitive, vulnerable, emotional, or subservient to others are feminine characteristics, so many guys are uncomfortable when their "soft" qualities are exposed to others. But manliness isn't only about toughening up, riding into battle, being brave and courageous, and being emotionless. The true definition of manliness is ancient, and it looks nothing like how people describe it. The Latin word for manliness is *virtus* (from which we get the English word "virtue"). Initially emphasizing bravery and courage, the Roman concept of *virtus* gradually expanded to include traits such as fortitude, industry, and duty.

Similarly, in ancient Greek, the word "manliness" (*andreia*) was used synonymously with "virtue" (*arete*). A man of *arete* realized his entire bodily, mental, and spiritual potential. Despite obstacles and difficulties, he accomplished his goals skillfully and left a meaningful and enduring legacy. So, for the Ancient Romans and Greeks, manliness meant living a life of virtue.

Society and culture have misled us about the definition of a real man. It portrays men as all about power, toughness, money, and women. Instead, a true man is one who exudes real masculinity and self-confidence. He is a man who is aware of his own thoughts and life goals and is not hesitant to speak up in support of his convictions. He concentrates on cultivating the qualities that will enable him to continue growing and becoming a better man at each new stage of his life to become the finest possible version of himself. Like the ancients, our philosophy of the modern man is straightforward: strive for virtue, honor, and perfection in all facets of life, realize your full potential as a man, and be the best version of yourself.

The word "beast" might come off as aggressive or violent. However, the "Beast Mode" we talk about in this book is far from this. Beast Mode is an attitude, a mentality, and a lifestyle. It is about adopting a disciplined and proactive mindset to bring out the best in yourself. Modern men are flooded with difficult circumstances, but unleashing your Beast Mode is going to help you handle these challenges and develop the work ethic that 99 percent of others lack. Developing your Beast Mode will require a combination of hard work, persistence, and a strong mentality. This book will introduce you to the habits, principles, and mindsets that are going to pave your path to success.

Beast Mode for the Modern Man is a book on men's wellness brimming with proven principles, strategies, and techniques that will help you become the man you always wanted to be. The illusion of needing excessive power, money, and sex has possessed and crippled most modern men. Therefore, men are at war with themselves daily, consumed by the rat race of life. This book will open your eyes and help you discover modern masculinity. You will learn all the right paradigms to become a true man, and it will help you learn practical ways to lead a happy, healthy life that you are proud of.

Our goal in writing this book is to enlighten you, to provide a path and direction for you to step more completely into your own authenticity, and to expand your capacity for caring for yourself. We have witnessed many men struggling because they are so cut off from the depths of their potential and have distanced themselves from the qualities that would allow them to have a life they love. The life of a modern man is anchored not in possessions but in the *essence* of who they are. This book is intended to honor such a life.

CHAPTER 1

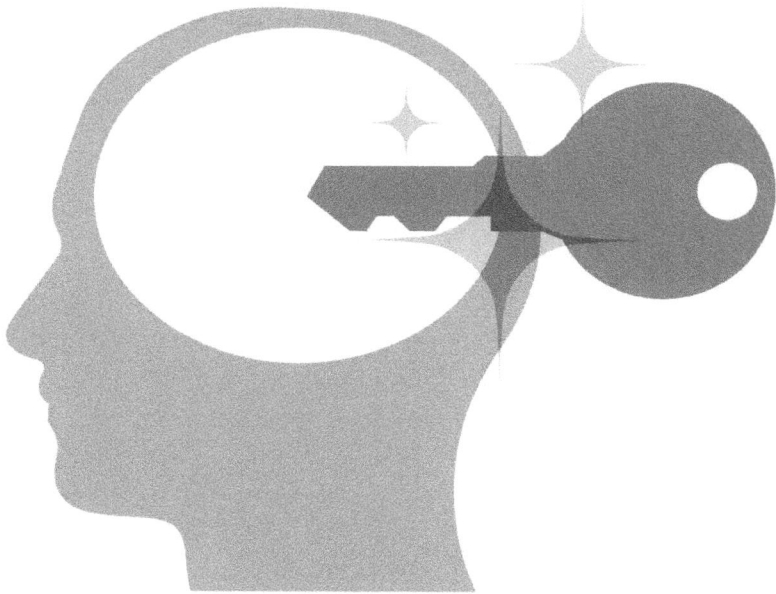

BREAKING
THE MYTHS

1

BREAKING THE MYTHS

We grew up with the notion that being a man meant projecting control and strength while guarding against showing any emotions that may imply softness or weakness. Our heroes were superheroes with super strengths and emotionally resolute movie characters. The media, television, and the whole of society have painted a distinct picture of men. And although we live in a confusing time when traditional values and gender roles are being flipped 180 degrees, there are certain misconceptions and prejudices still deeply ingrained in our society.

"What makes a man?" There are so many false beliefs, unhealthy expectations, and even lies that circle around this question. These misconceptions are detrimental to our health, our relationships, and, most importantly, our happiness. These stereotypes are passed from generation to generation because most fathers do not teach their kids what true masculinity is. Instead, they teach their kids to give in to the fake and harmful prejudice of society. In this chapter, we debunk some of the myths men deal with and discuss how to solve these stereotypes.

. . .

EMOTIONS ARE FOR THE WEAK

Jacob was only five years old when his parents bought him his first bicycle. He was super excited. He took his bicycle for a spin and, in no time at all, fell off and hurt his knees. Just like every other five-year-old, his natural response was to cry. Jacob's father saw the tears filling his eyes and, being the parent he was, he reacted instinctively. He didn't want to watch his young son crying. His exact words:

"Don't cry. Boys don't cry!"

Despite Jacob's mediocre memory, his father's phrase has stuck with him to this day, deeply and strongly. As he got older, Jacob assumed a man's tears were a sign of weakness. He needed to overcome shortcomings such as these if he wanted to be a man.

Nobody should blame Jacob's father because this is perhaps the same treatment he received from *his* father. Society created these paradigms. The Alpha Male is one who has a heart of stone with little to no emotions and does not display reactions to physical or mental trauma. In the eyes of the world, emotion is a sign of femininity and weakness.

The idea that men should always portray their power over their emotions is the foundation of the myth of weakness. But the reality is men's physical and mental health suffers greatly as a result of the pressure to suppress their emotions. Men must constantly worry that even a "chink in the armor" of their self-confidence, independence, and assurance would make them look weak.

The majority of men conceal and hide their emotions as they are socially obligated to be "protectors."

Whether you believe it or not, men have a complete spectrum of emotional experiences that influence us in ways we don't typically speak about. As society changes, dialogue around this stigma is shifting as networks of men make it possible to discuss difficulties without passing judgment. However, I would take one step further and state that being vulnerable is a sign of strength rather than weakness. This is not an opinion but a fact.

Withholding our emotions does nothing other than create a toxic mental and emotional environment. If we shut all our trash in a windowless room, eventually, it will smell and rot. The same can be said of men's emotions. To relieve the strain, we must air things out. We're not advocating sobbing uncontrollably through every Hallmark movie, but understanding that emotions are not a sign of weakness. Vulnerability is a sign of courage, no matter the gender.

MEN MUST HAVE IT ALL TOGETHER

What does a man say when everything in his life is going south?

"I'll figure it out."

Does he actually figure it out? Well, not always. It's no secret that men have ego problems when it comes to asking for assistance. But why? For most men, seeking support from others means they don't have it all together. Men believe this inability reflects their weaknesses and exposes their flaws in front of others.

Men have a natural tendency to present as problem solvers. They like to figure things out, find solutions, and get things done. But they also have a very big ego, one that builds on the stereotype that men should have all the answers, all the knowledge, or at least have the capacity to figure it out on their own. They have these false assumptions that if they require assistance, there must be something wrong with them.

Men find it challenging to seek aid since they don't want to look needy in front of their friends and family. We all probably know someone who gets lost in cities but won't ask for directions. Someone who will spend hours tinkering with a device before finally calling in an expert. The origin of this behavior comes from the "should" statements that permeate society.

"Men should have it all figured out…"

"Men should be able to deal with it on their own…"

3

"Men should be able to handle anything that comes their way..."

Our lives change, and our society progresses, but the stereotypes remain the same.

Society expects men to abide by some fictitious norms. However, these expectations are overwhelming and burdensome to their physical and mental health.

Whether we acknowledge it or not, everyone needs help from someone at one point or another. It is a natural part of being a human. So, we must not do this to ourselves. Remember that reaching our full potential is not something that we can achieve alone. We need help, and there is nothing to be ashamed of.

SIZE MATTERS

According to a study published in 2006 by Psychology of Men and Masculinity, 85 percent said that they were very satisfied with their male partner's penis size when asked. Ironically, though, only 45 percent of men felt satisfied and adequate in their size. This research should easily debunk the "size matters" myth, as it's more psychological than physical. However, the answer is simple. It does not! So, if partners are satisfied, why do men feel so insecure?

"Toxic masculinity" refers to a collection of societal messages that pressurize men to behave macho, repress their emotions, and lean into masculine characteristics. Related to this is the belief that a larger penis correlates with increased manliness and virility. Cultural cues—and popular media on TV and in men's magazines— regularly link men's penis size to masculinity, increasing men's anxieties about their own.

Another aspect that fuels this myth is the unrealistic depiction of bodies in porn, which often shows men's penises as substantially bigger than average. This engraves the misconception that a man's penis should ideally be that large. Additionally, women's exaggerated sexual reactions to highly endowed men in these adult films also influence the belief that women significantly desire larger penises.

The size of your penis is not as important as how you use it, your communication skills, and how well you pay attention to your partner's satisfaction. If you are self-conscious about the size of your penis, you are not alone; almost every guy is insecure about it. But keep in mind that good sex does not specifically include penetration, and your masculinity is not tied to your penis size.

MEN'S VALUE SHOULD BE DETERMINED BY HOW MUCH THEY EARN

For the majority of men, the stresses of work originate from two sources:

- the necessity to support their families, and
- the desire to succeed at something.

However, all too often, society blends the responsibility and identity of men. A man is not his job. A person's duties cannot be intermingled with his identity. This also applies to women but men are traditionally defined by their occupations more often.

As men grow up, they learn to be competitive; they learn that their participation in the rat race is important for maintaining their self-respect. In our society, a man's occupation and income are indicators of his worth. These are what determine the respect and love he will receive. It's no wonder men place such an inappropriate emphasis on materialism when under this intense pressure.

Power is the ability to take action, bring about meaningful change, and force our will on our surroundings, whether they are internal or external. Men are taught from childhood that the only way to establish authority and exercise power is to have money, wealth, and fame. Without it, you are of little to no significance.

"Only women, children, and dogs are loved unconditionally. A man is only loved under the condition that he provides something." – Chris Rock

Whether you agree or disagree with the quote, this is a misconception that constantly haunts the mental health of men. This misconception not only fosters detrimental gender roles but massively burdens men with unrealistic expectations. Men are complex, multifaceted individuals. They must be respected for their abilities, talents, and contributions in a variety of spheres of life, not only in their careers. Their value is greater than their bank account and social status.

MEN ONLY WANT SEX

"Guys literally only want one thing."

This was Tweeted by a girl back in 2017. It garnered a lot of attention from the netizens, especially female ones (Loveific, n.d.).

The "one thing" the tweet refers to is obviously sex. Although mostly thrown out as a joke, this illustrates how society as a whole promotes the idea that men are robots with basic programming, and everything they do is focused on their next sexual conquest. It is notions like these that shape the cultural context of today, influencing how men and women interact with one another.

The idea that men only want sex closes discussions without addressing the crucial topic of why men do not want to commit in the first place. The simple answer is that most guys don't have a problem being loyal to one woman. (Yes, I said *most* men.) But men don't want to spend money on relationships that don't enrich their lives or make them feel fulfilled. There are obviously exceptions, and there are examples of men who do only want "one thing." But exceptions can rarely be used as solid examples to represent the majority.

In movies, TV shows, and media, men are portrayed as reckless and impulsive when it comes to relationships. However, in reality, most men choose their partners with considerably more contemplation and caution. Men will probably have a lot of unsuccessful hookups, relationships, and situation-ships while looking for the right partner and, as is often the case, many will have their advances turned down by women. However, the opposite is also true, and many men will reject women they believe are incompatible. So, when feelings are hurt and hearts are broken, the women who were turned down will believe and impose the fact that "men only want one thing."

This is unfortunate and reinforces a false perception of men's motivations and what they want from women. But if the myth that men want only one thing is wrong, what do they really want?

It might be challenging to condense the desires of all 3.5 billion men on earth into a single sentence. However, it is possible to create broad guidelines to characterize the preferences of the majority of men.

To put it simply: men want stability and consistency. These two words might signify various things to different people, but the underlying idea is always the same. Stability, in this case, refers to a man feeling safe enough to invest himself in a relationship. A guy seeks assurance that his efforts won't be in vain in the event of a partner's abrupt attitude shift, particularly one that is beyond his control. Each man may define security differently, but it mostly refers to having unwavering support during difficult times, emotional reciprocation, genuine interest in their projects, etc.

We all change, and there is no true stability. But what men really want to know is whether a woman's core qualities will still be there ten or twenty years down the line. So, if there is any single thing that men want, it isn't sex. It's the same thing every other person wants—to love and be loved in return.

MEN HAVE IT EASY

This is obviously a very contradictory opinion because very few women will agree that this is a myth. There are reasons why a woman might feel this way:

- Men need mere moments to get ready.
- It's socially acceptable for men to go bald naturally.
- Men do not menstruate.
- Men do not have to go through childbirth.

The list goes on…

To some extent, they are correct. We have it easy when it comes to societal grooming expectations; we have it easy when it comes to reproduction; we have it easy since we do not have to go through the monthly suffering of period cramps. However, it is not always a bed of roses. Rather, men just experience difficulty differently and in different ways.

Men's struggles are more typically mental and financial than physical. Obviously, this is no comparison of who has it easier. Both genders have their fair share of troubles that are completely different from one another.

It's not a competition or a debate on who has it easier; it's a matter of raising awareness and compassion.

Throughout history, there have been many misconceptions about the male gender. These myths are multifactorial and caused by numerous things, including long-held gender stereotypes, the underrepresentation of men in media and cultural narratives, historical context, fear of vulnerability, and patriarchal systems. Harmful beliefs about masculinity result from these, often imposing inflexible expectations about the behavior, emotions, and interests of men. The idea that men should be strong, emotionless, and in control is rooted in historical contexts in which masculinity was associated with power and dominance. To establish a more equal and inclusive society for all genders, we must refute and debunk these beliefs. Everyone should be free to be themselves by dismantling gender norms and accepting the variety of masculine expressions.

CHAPTER 2

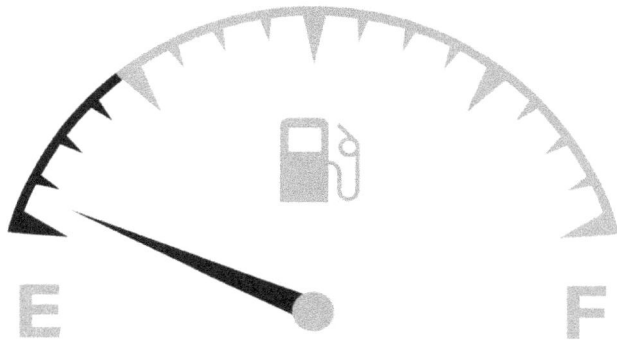

LIFESTYLE OF THE MODERN MAN

2

LIFESTYLE OF THE MODERN MAN

There are so many social stereotypes revolving around men, but social stigmata are not the only issues men face today. There are numerous critical aspects affecting the overall quality of a man's life. Everyone has their fair share of ups and downs, but the problem when it comes to men's problems is that they are rarely addressed. Many scoff or roll their eyes at even the notion of being asked to empathize with the struggles of today's men. It is important we internalize and investigate these problems and find solutions to improve the physical, mental, and emotional well-being of men.

Despite the constant presence of privilege, men tend to endure their own unique set of restrictions, which limit what it means to be a man and how a man expresses himself. This is particularly true for those who are members of marginalized groups. As a guy struggles to overcome issues, he is met with seemingly insurmountable difficulties. In this chapter, we discuss the pain points of the modern man's life and how unleashing the Beast Mode can bring out the best in you.

OVERWORKED AND BURNED OUT

The hustle culture is real. You will notice this all over the internet. People now boast about how many hours they have spent working as if they'll get an Olympic gold medal for it. Social media influencers are constantly trying to tell others how working "REALLY hard" has helped them live the life of their dreams. In addition to all this, technology keeps us in constant touch with our work.

Remember when people worked their nine-to-five job and then went home without having to worry about what their boss was doing, thinking, or planning? Those days are long gone. Our bosses can always reach us thanks to the mini offices we keep in our pockets, our smartphones. Even when enjoying a vacation in the Canary Islands, you now have to answer calls and emails that come your way. You don't leave work at the office; you bring it home. We should not be cursing technology for this because we ourselves have created this culture; we chose to participate in the rat race.

We're not trying to pick your flaws here. It's not just you; it's everyone you see around you. It's the pressure to succeed in school, the pressure to get into a good college, the pressure to get a high-earning job, and the pressure to earn a six-figure salary. There is nothing wrong with hard work. We are all for it. But this is getting out of control.

For some people, the persistent need to be in charge, have control over all situations, and to be busy is a sign of masculinity. Even as gender roles become more flexible, men are still often held to an unjustified standard. Women are sometimes the subject of articles about burnout, but never men. According to a 2021 study, 52 percent of American employees were burned out, up 9 percent from pre-Covid figures (Nelson 2022). After the inception of the Covid pandemic, longer working hours became one major reason for men's burnout worldwide.

Working sixty to eighty hours is not healthy, nor is it sustainable. Depression, anxiety, insomnia, and excessive drinking are all symptoms that men are pushing themselves toward to deny that they are overworked. In a society moving quicker than ever, it seems that men, in particular, are always on the go, which may cause serious health issues. According to recent research by the Canadian Men's Health Foundation, contemporary men may really be putting themselves in danger of dying young due to burnout and stress (Majaski 2019).

We held interviews with employees at a global strategy consulting firm with a strong presence. The company we studied provides consulting services across a range of specialties and works in small teams to finish client projects. In the office, consultants are expected to be ready for any last-minute weekend and late work assignments, as well as overnight travel to client locations. Here is what one employee told us:

"Sometimes, I have to take calls on Sunday evenings. Sometimes, I have to make calls early on Saturdays. So, the weekend does not remain a weekend. I simply must be there when the customer requires it of me. You don't really have the freedom to decline an invitation to consulting or the professional services sector as a whole. If you are unable to attend, it is most likely because you have another customer meeting scheduled at the same time. You simply cannot say that you cannot be there because your son has a baseball game."

This gives you a picture of what it means to be a man today.

But the worst part is not the physical or mental symptoms of burnout; it is the loss of confidence. When you are that burned out, living off coffee and fast food and only getting exercise from commuting to and from your vehicle, you will not be at your best. And when you cannot perform, your job will start to suffer. This is when you start to have negative thoughts about yourself.

What's wrong with me?

Why am I falling behind?

How is everyone handling the same thing so much better than me?

You start to believe that you are not working hard enough and that you need to put in more effort. Your confidence is ruined, and you start giving twice the effort. The cycle goes on forever.

BEAST MODE LIFESTYLE TO MANAGE BURNOUT

Burnout can happen to anyone. All of us have faced it in some parts of our lives. You become exhausted, overburdened, and unrested. Consequently, you get fatigued and have sporadic emotional outbursts, responding irrationally to even the smallest inconveniences. Pushing yourself to the limit can be detrimental to your relationships and physical and mental well-being. If you are suffering from burnout, you need to harness the Beast Mode lifestyle and mindset to counteract the effects and combat the negativity that comes with it.

But before we talk about managing burnout, you need to have a good understanding of why you're facing it in the first place. Here are five common reasons:

1. **Working toward something:** Men are goal-oriented. You probably don't like the idea of lagging behind others, right?. You put in seventy to eighty hours a week to get noticed. After working several years in the company, you are on the brink of a raise or promotion, and you want to give it your all to accomplish this.
2. **Working to avoid something:** Work can sometimes be your getaway. It can distract you from all the other problems you have in your life, such as a failing relationship, a broken family, a financial crisis, and so on. You hate to leave the office and end your working day because it means you have to return to all your problems at home.
3. **The Hustle Culture:** A classic one for sure; "Since everyone else is doing it, I should too." Some offices reward this culture of working until burnout. Workplaces will

deliver meals with the notion you will work far into the evening or will give raises to those who arrive early and leave late. These and many other bullshit traditions make no sense and drive you to work long hours and, eventually, to burnout.

4. **Inability to say "NO":** If the above reasons do not apply to you, face it, you are a people-pleaser. You want to be liked by your manager, coworkers, and clients. You work from home, take on more responsibilities, and even when it's uncomfortable, you agree to fill in for your colleagues. When you are this accessible, it is normal for others to take advantage of you and make you work long hours.

5. **Being a perfectionist:** Perhaps the problem is not others; the problem is you. Are you a perfectionist? Are you are adding to your own workload by constantly editing, revising, and rewriting material. Do you lack the skills necessary to unwind and feel at ease while working?

We are pretty sure that you fall into one of the above five categories. Now that you understand the reasons behind your overworking, it will be much easier to implement the Beast Mode lifestyle and chip away at your bad habits, which are causing the detrimental effects of burnout. The whole idea of unleashing the beast in you is to rise above norms and stigmata like a phoenix from the ashes.

It might be hard to see the end of the tunnel once burnout sets in. You might experience extreme emotional exhaustion and despair; you might experience a sense of hopelessness and lack of drive to continue. But don't worry. Implementing the following techniques and principles into your life can drastically change the way you feel about yourself, work and your career.

Reframe your mindset: Of course, the first suggestion is to leave your job (if you hate it) and look for one you love. However, this is impractical for many. If you can't quit your job, you *can* choose to change a few things about it. But what?

Even in the most mundane jobs, it's possible to find a way your work benefits others. Pay attention to the parts of your job that you do like, even if it's the morning coffee or the lunch break conversations. Alter the way you see your work, and you may re-establish a feeling of direction and control. Many individuals who experience burnout hyper-focus on the negative aspects of their jobs or roles. This may increase burnout by making the work or position feel even more difficult, unpleasant, and irritating. The 'Blue Car Syndrome' suggests if someone says to you "don't look for the Blue Car" chances are, you will see blue cars everywhere. Similarly, by focusing on the negative aspects of your job, you will attract more of it. Conversely, if you focus on the positive aspects, you will attract more of that. What you focus on, you will get more of. Choice is yours.

If your job is just boring and there's no good you can think about it, consider making friends. Yes, strong relationships at work may lessen boredom and stave off burnout symptoms. A difficult or unfulfilling job may be stressful but having friends to laugh with throughout the day can help. It can make you feel better that you are not alone in a hellhole, but have friends who have got your back.

In addition to this, if your job seems unfulfilling, search for fulfillment and significance in other areas of your life, such as your friends, family, hobbies, or volunteer work. Pay attention to the aspects of your life that make you happy and avoid thinking of those that do not.

Furthermore, consider upskilling or moving into a new role or department in the company. Consider dusting off that crazy business idea that you have put on the shelf for years! Entrepreneurs are born when they venture outside the comfort zone and take action in the face of adversity and challenges.

Turn to other people: When facing burnout, the future seems gloomy. It becomes almost impossible to have the energy for self-care, let alone to take the initiative to help yourself. But there is a lot you can do to salvage yourself from this situation. Social interaction is nature's remedy for stress, and speaking face-to-face with a patient listener is one of the quickest methods for relaxing. Your conversation partner does not have to cure your worries; they just have to be a good listener, someone who will pay close attention without getting side tracked or passing judgment.

The Beast Mode lifestyle implies you will be vulnerable and embrace this vulnerability. There is no reason to hide your feelings of burnout. Instead, reach out to your spouse, family, friends, and anybody dear to you. You won't be a burden to others if you open up. It will only solidify your connection since most friends and family will be touched that you trust them enough to tell them about your insecurities. Talking about your exhaustion will make you feel lighter and will help you discover new ways of coping with work.

While it's super important to make friends at your workplace, it's also important to avoid negative people. It's common for energy-draining vampires who exude nothing but negativity to roam your office. Spending time with these individuals, who only complain and nag, will bring your mood down. You don't have to confront them; avoiding them does not make you weak. If you have no option but to work with them, try to avoid small talk and make sure you do not discuss anything personal with them.

Reevaluate your priorities: Burnout is a sign that something important in your life is *dysfunctional*. If you are experiencing this, you need to spend some time reflecting on your aspirations and desires. Ask yourself, are you skipping out on something that matters to you deeply? This may be a good time to slow down and allow yourself some space to ponder and rediscover what really makes you happy.

While it's important to strive for greatness and exceed expectations, it's equally important to establish healthy boundaries. Like transitioning from working hard to working smart, setting boundaries is crucial for maintaining a sustainable and balanced lifestyle. It's essential to recognize and respect your personal limitations, including how much work you can handle and how much time you need to recharge. Learning to decline requests that don't align with your priorities can be achieved by following the "Hell Yeah," or "N.O. capital N, capital O" rule, which encourages you to only commit to opportunities that truly excite you.

If you have doubts about doing something, don't do it. Only take part in things that give you the notion of "Hell Yeah." Otherwise, develop the guts to say "NO," and in your mind, say "capital N, capital O," which will empower you with your decision. Keep in mind that saying "no" frees you up to say "yes" to the commitments you want to make.

As mentioned previously, one of the reasons we cannot detach ourselves from work is our constant relationship with technology. It is important you take time away from electronics and technology every day. Decide on a time you will entirely unplug. Put your laptop away, switch off your phone, and refrain from checking social media or email at all. Utilize this time to enrich your social life, gain knowledge by reading books, develop a new skill, or give time to self-care. You can also think about taking up new fun projects or pick up your old interests again. Choose hobbies that rejuvenate and fulfill you. This is your time to put back into you.

Additionally, you could look toward relaxation practices, such as yoga, meditation, deep breathing or adult coloring books. We will talk more about these in the next chapter.

Rather than waiting to put out flames, it is preferable to prevent burnout entirely or to deal with it as soon as you see symptoms arise. When burned out, your body and spirit make you pay attention to them. Finding and maintaining your natural pace of life is the key to preventing burnout and recovering from it. Remember that resilience is not about how you survive but how you refuel. Using the Beast Mode strategies above, you will supercharge yourself to prevent burnout and reach your ultimate potential.

STRESS, ANXIETY, AND DEPRESSION

Men do not want to look weak. They want to portray that they are strong, independent, and able to tolerate any suffering that comes their way. Men might often put off getting any form of help to preserve that image of themselves. That is why you will notice that men find it extremely challenging to admit when they are having mental health problems. Around forty million people in America suffer from anxiety disorders, the most prevalent mental ailment according to the Anxiety and Depression Association of America (*Anxiety Disorders – Facts & Statistics*, n.d.) Despite men and women experiencing anxiety, depression, and stress equally, men present their symptoms quite differently.

This difference in symptoms and expression is due to the social and biological factors that influence a man's coping mechanisms. Anxiety and depression can often present as:

- anger,
- irritability,
- insomnia,
- strained relationships,
- Overeating or undereating
- substance abuse, and so on.

Instead of expressing their anxiety or depression, men are more likely to exhibit aggressive behavior, which is regarded as more acceptable in society. They frequently downplay and avoid expressing negative emotions and thus may often burst into anger. You will notice how depression manifests differently in new dads than in new moms. Men who experience perinatal depression and anxiety may withdraw from their families, become irate and angry, have trouble falling asleep, and abuse alcohol or drugs.

One in eight men experience anxiety and/or depression at some stage in their life, but fewer than half of them take medication or get professional help. Even more concerning is the strong correlation between anxiety disorders and suicide attempts. In the

United States, suicide rates are rising, and men are more than three times as likely to commit suicide than women (McClain, 2019). This is alarming, and it is high time men changed their lifestyle and mindset about mental health to break from its shackles.

The reasons behind anxiety and depression in men are similar to those behind their tendency to become overworked and overburdened. Four reasons that frequently come up are:

1. Constantly being connected online.
2. Trying to do too much in too little time.
3. Not having tools for prioritization.
4. Poor stress-release mechanisms.

While the reasons are the same, avoiding burnout and avoiding anxiety and depression is not the same; one is related to your professional life, and the other takes you down completely. So how does a man implement the Beast Mode lifestyle to deal with the anxiety and stress of the modern world? What coping mechanisms does he use to survive the everyday struggle?

BEAST MODE LIFESTYLE TO MANAGE STRESS, ANXIETY AND DEPRESSION

The Beast Mode lifestyle is not going to tell you to "MAN UP." Harnessing toxic masculinity is not ideal for coping with anxiety or stress. This bad advice has pushed men to such extreme health conditions already. As we saw above, men are already committing suicide at alarming rates. It's not the time for toxic masculinity. Men need real, actionable advice and solutions to help ease their anxiety and depression. It's time to help you leave your misery behind and live a life you love.

Ease up with expectations: More often than we know, our own expectations contribute the greatest to our anxiety. It's likely that you have high expectations of yourself. You demand to become the best in what you do whenever and however you do it. But these high expectations, at least to some extent, are a major contributor to your anxiety.

When we demand too much of ourselves, we push our bodies and minds past their limits. Many of us who strive for such excellence often fall victim to pushing too far by establishing standards that are unrealizable, inflexible, or impossible to meet. This positions you for failure, disappointment, and a poor opinion of yourself.

Expectations create pressure and anticipation about our future goals, events, and personal performance. When we set the bar high, we set ourselves up for a specific outcome. And if things don't go as we expect them to, it shatters our confidence and makes us insecure.

Expectations are made up of neural circuits in our brains. These neural circuits are developed based on our experiences. Each experience of pain and pleasure connects neurons that control our expectations about future pleasure and suffering. Although we may not realize it, expectations guide our attempts to make sense of the world. Our brains constantly scan our environment and absorb more data than they can handle. Our brains then create predictions about the next piece of information they will receive to make sense of the information overload and search for a fitting sensory input.

An expectation is not a conscious thought but a trickle of electricity that passes through a conduit created by prior experience. When there is a match between the expected and the reality, our brain releases dopamine, the neurotransmitter that gives you "good" feelings. On the contrary, if the reality and expectations do not match, cortisol is released from our body, which is responsible for creating the sensation of anxiety.

When we encounter a new experience that doesn't fit with what we already know, we face a decision. We can stick with what we already believe and follow the same mental path we've always taken, or we can try to think differently and create a new neural pathway. It can be hard to create new mental pathways because our brains are wired to follow the same well-worn paths we've taken before. This means we often end up sticking with what we know instead of trying something new.

I know what you're thinking: *"Shut up with the boring brain chemistry. Tell us what we should do to lower our expectations!"*

The reason explaining brain chemistry is important is that I need you to realize that expectations are bodily responses to experiences. They do not define who we are, nor do they reflect our values or ethics. There is no point in being driven by expectations. Instead, we must be driven by the goals and dreams we set for ourselves to objectively keep in line with our values.

Here are some questions to help you out:

- Are the expectations I have set for myself actually achievable?
- What part of my expectations can I control?
- Are my expectations my own, or are they influenced by my co-workers, friends or family?
- Am I being ungrateful for everything I already have?

The answer to these questions will help you understand yourself better. Remember, the Beast Mode lifestyle is not about having no expectations; it is about establishing attainable goals. Having realistic expectations that are your own and aren't influenced by the people around you will help you feel better overall. You will feel less stressed and more in control.

Focus on things you can change: Often, our anxiety and depression originate from worrying about events that have not yet occurred or may never happen. Despite the uncertainties in our lives, it is important to keep in mind that we can always choose how we respond to a circumstance, no matter how difficult it is.

There is a famous quote by the stoic Seneca:

"We suffer more in imagination than in reality."

We need to prioritize the present instead of worrying about things that may or may not happen. Due to the amount of information we are fed by social media and the internet, our brain is continuously switching contexts within a fraction of a second. This shifts our focus from one thing to another and does not let us enjoy the present. We become fixated on unrealistic and imaginary worries about the future.

The Beast Mode lifestyle encourages us to live in the moment, meaning we must be aware and mindful of what we are doing now. Instead of worrying, you need to focus on the now to change the future. The secret to a healthy and happy life is the ability to focus on things you can change and avoid the things you cannot. This keeps you grounded and connected to yourself and everything around you, reduces your stress and ruminating, and helps in your battle against anxiety.

While staying present may seem like fashionable advice popular all over the internet, it is a way of life supported by sound research. Being present and aware may make us happier, more able to manage discomfort, lessen stress and its bad effects on our health, and make us better able to handle unpleasant emotions like fear and rage.

Practice deep and focused breathing: What's the first thing people say to you when you say you are feeling anxious? "RELAX." For most people, relaxation is watching TV and lying down on your couch after a difficult day. However, this type of relaxation doesn't do much to lessen the negative impacts of anxiety or stress. To effectively combat anxiety, it's important to activate the body's natural relaxation mechanisms.

One way that we recommend is the 4–7–8 breathing technique. This was developed by Dr. Andrew Weil and is based on an ancient yogic technique called pranayama. This technique is designed to increase the amount of oxygen that reaches your vital organs and tissues, starting from your lungs and spreading throughout your body to relax you deeply. The 4–7–8 technique works by having you hold your breath for a specific period of time, which can help your body rehydrate its oxygen supply.

When anxious, our fight-or-flight response is stimulated. With the help of relaxation techniques like 4–7–8 breathing, we can inhibit this response and restore our body's equilibrium. This breathing technique will compel your mind and body to concentrate on controlling your breath rather than reliving your worries.

Here's how the process works:

1. Choose a comfortable spot to sit or lay down in.
2. Be careful of your posture, particularly at first. Lying down is optimal for this method.
3. Let your lips separate and exhale through your mouth using a whooshing motion.
4. Seal your lips and breathe quietly through your nose for four seconds.
5. Hold your breath for seven seconds.
6. Repeat the previous whooshing exhalation for eight seconds.

(Legg and Dasgupta, 2018)

A fresh cycle of breath begins after you inhale once more. Practice this pattern for a full four breaths. The most important aspect of this technique is holding the breath (held for seven seconds).

Practicing abdominal breathing like this for twenty to thirty minutes daily can greatly lessen your anxiety and stress. Deep breathing activates your parasympathetic nervous system and makes you feel calmer than normal. By focusing on your breathing, you will feel more at ease with your body and shun your body's anxiety responses.

The journey through anxiety is individual to you, so it might take time to find what works best for you. We encourage you to try the breathing exercise above and be patient and kind to yourself. If your anxiety affects the quality of your life, do not be afraid or ashamed of getting professional help. Anxiety, unlike a broken leg where one's crutches are visible, is not seen by the naked eye. It doesn't mean it does not exist. Remember that everyone needs help at some time in their lives.

SLEEP DEPRIVATION IN MEN

While we may not realize this, our physical and mental well-being is tied to the amount and quality of sleep we get each night. Research suggests that, on average, women are more likely to get more sleep than men, and this is perhaps influenced by men's responsibilities toward work and family (Robards and Troy, 2023). Although the American Academy of Sleep Medicine advises getting more than seven hours of sleep each night, a survey revealed that nearly a third (29.2 percent) of men slept for less than six hours each night (Robards and Troy, 2023).

Sleep is not a luxury; it is a necessity so often overlooked. Scarily, sleep deprivation may have detrimental long-term impacts on your health even if you don't toss and turn every night. According to a study, sleep researchers have concluded that having fewer than six to eight hours of sleep each night increases your chance of dying young by as much as 12 percent (Butler, 2018).

When we have a busy day, our brains need time to consolidate memories, process emotions, and refresh themselves using the glymphatic system. This happens when we sleep. When we don't get enough sleep, our brains cannot complete these processes, which can make us feel tired and sleepy. One sign of sleep deprivation is relying on a lot of coffee to get through the day. Although caffeine can temporarily mask the effects of sleep deprivation, once the caffeine wears off, we may feel even more exhausted because the processes our brain must go through while sleeping, such as consolidating memories, are incomplete. Therefore, if we don't get enough sleep, it makes us drowsy.

For many men, sleep remains at the bottom of their list. They prioritize other forms of self-care instead. Some even consider sleep to be a waste of time. These false beliefs prevent men from benefiting from the strength of a rested mind and body. Along with nutrition and exercise, sleep is one of the pillars of health. The more you put into your sleep, the greater return you will experience in all other areas of your life. It is anything but a waste of time. During sleep, your body actively recharges and prepares you for the next day. When you get a good night's sleep, you will feel, think, and function better and will be able to make the most of your time and energy the next day.

The following are some signs that you are not getting the sleep you need:

- You experience daytime fatigue and a lack of energy.
- You have trouble concentrating.
- You lack motivation and struggle to "get moving."
- You often become angry, grumpy, or irritated.
- You start to doze off while you are in a meeting, driving, or sitting idly at your desk.

Keeping a hectic schedule is a feature of modern life. Men, in particular, may find themselves juggling many obligations such as a job, family, and social activities, which are judged more important than sleep and therefore exhaust a man's time and cause him to stay up later than he should.

In addition to having a busy life, men often get inadequate sleep due to the notion of what it means to be a man. A 2021 research article from the Journal of the Association for Consumer Research investigates a potential connection between sleep and masculinity. The research suggests that men who sleep less are perceived as more masculine. Also, men who sleep less are seen to be more favorable by society (Robards, 2023). Our work culture and our society glorify the idea of sleeplessness, endangering our health and safety.

Being sleep deprived is not something to be proud of. Lack of sleep affects your thinking, emotions, memory, and even your capacity to make moral judgments. Workplace sleepiness and weariness result in decreased productivity, trouble thinking creatively, and increased chances of mistakes and/or accidents.

While there are people who consciously deprive themselves of sleep, there are others whose life circumstances force them to cut down. Although you can't control uncertain circumstances, it's important to remember that getting a good night's sleep can be one of the best ways to deal with complex emotional situations. When you sleep well, your mind can process your emotions and help you get rid of negative feelings. This can help you wake up feeling more positive and ready to tackle the next day.

BEAST MODE LIFESTYLE TO MANAGE SLEEP DEPRIVATION

As mentioned above, many factors could be interfering with your sleep. You might not always have control over these things, but you *can* choose to adopt habits that encourage more sleep and protect you from the vicious cycle of sleep deprivation. Here are some tips to change your lifestyle for the better:

- **Follow a sleep schedule:** You can't even guess how important this is. Create a sleep schedule and follow it strictly. Go to bed and wake up at the same hour every single morning and evening. (Yes, weekends, too.) Consistency strengthens the sleep-wake cycle in your body. If you cannot sleep after twenty minutes of lying down, get out of bed and relax. Try reading a book or listening to soothing music. You could even try some adult coloring books, which help promote stress relief and relaxation by calming the fear center of the brain. When you feel exhausted, go back to bed. Repeat as many times as necessary but keep your sleep and wake time consistent.

- **Increase bright-light exposure during the day:** Our body has an internal clock known as the circadian rhythm. This impacts our hormones, body, and brain, keeping us alert and letting our body know when it's time to sleep. Your circadian rhythm is kept healthy through exposure to natural sunshine or strong light throughout the day. This increases both the quality and length of the night's sleep as well as daily energy. According to studies, exposure to bright daylight throughout the afternoon lengthened and increased the quality of insomniacs' sleep. Moreover, 83 percent less time was needed to fall asleep (Anderson, n.d.). Try to expose yourself to sunshine each day. If this is not possible, invest in a device or light bulbs that produce bright artificial light.
- **Reduce blue light exposure in the evening:** While exposure to light in the daytime is preferred, light exposure at nighttime has the reverse impact. Blue light alters your circadian cycle and deceives your brain into believing it is sunlight. This lowers your levels of sleep chemicals, like melatonin, which promote relaxation and deep sleep. The light produced by devices such as cell phones and computers is the most harmful. Here are a few things you can do about it:

o Wear glasses to block blue light.

o Download apps like Flux to block blue light coming from your computer.

o Install a blue-light-filtering app on your phone.

o Stop looking at screens two hours before going to bed.

- **Stop consuming caffeine late in the day:** Ninety percent of Americans drink caffeine, and a single cup of coffee can improve your concentration and energy levels (Johnson, n.d.). But it is also true that caffeine stimulates your nervous system when ingested later in the day, which can prevent your body from properly relaxing at night. The levels of caffeine in your blood can remain high for six to eight hours after drinking coffee. Therefore, as noted in the article "Actions of caffeine in the brain with special reference to factors that contribute to its widespread use" by Fredholm and others, it is not advised to consume a lot of coffee after three or four p.m., particularly if you are sensitive to caffeine or have difficulties falling asleep. If you simply cannot survive without coffee late in the day, why not try decaf?

- **Optimize your environment:** This is something so many individuals ignore. Our surroundings play a significant role in the habits we create for ourselves. This is a concept James Clear discusses elaborately in his book *Atomic Habits*. When you create a favorable environment in which to perform a routine, you are more likely to follow through with it. And when you perform the routine regularly, that is when it turns into a habit. A good night's sleep is dependent on the bedroom setting and atmosphere. These elements include the following: temperature, sound, outside illumination, furniture placement, etc. Reduce external noise and artificial lighting from things like alarm clocks in your bedroom to the absolute minimum. Another way to enhance your sleeping environment is by using white noise. White noise contains every frequency within the range of human hearing, which creates a steady and consistent background sound that can help drown out other noises and instill calmness. This can be especially helpful if you live in a noisy area or have trouble sleeping due to external sounds.

- Ensure that your bedroom is a peaceful, comfortable, tidy, and pleasurable space. In addition, make sure you have a comfortable mattress, pillow, and bed. Make the experience a good one so that you enjoy the process of falling asleep instead of simply going to sleep because you have to.

Manage worries: One thing that might be keeping you up late at night is anxiety about the future. So, what can you do about this anxiety? Use the 4–7–8 breathing technique to calm yourself down. Relaxation techniques are proven to enhance the quality of your sleep. In addition to the breathing technique, try visualizing, listening to calming music, reading, having a hot bath, meditating, or using adult coloring books to calm yourself down for a good night's sleep. Test out several techniques to see which one suits you the best.

Overall, the number one thing is to understand the importance of sleep and prioritize it above other things in life. Implementing these tips can help you improve the quality and quantity of the sleep you get, but if you do not prioritize your sleep, you will end up back where you were. It is important to take these tips seriously if you truly want to live your life to the best of its potential.

HAVING NO TIME

When a man says he has no time, it is not that he is extremely busy, it is just that he has poor time management skills and is unable to cope with his responsibilities. Generally speaking, men want more time. They want to improve in their careers, find time for fitness, spend time with their families, partners, and children, or pursue their passions and hobbies while also developing social lives and new relationships. Doing all this can be overwhelming, but a man's got to do what a man's got to do.

Do you feel overwhelmingly busy? Like there isn't enough time in the day, and your schedule is just getting longer and longer? Yes, we have all been there. But the reality is most people who say they are too busy are doing it to themselves. We can always choose what we do with our time and how we spend it. Therefore, the way we use time is linked to the decisions we make. Our attitude toward time is also important, and instead of continuously blaming the clock, we should first address the elephant in the room; our psychology of time.

Have you wondered why time seems to fly when you are having fun but seems to drag by when you're not? That's not only you; that's all of us. One paper, examining studies of workplace happiness from 2011–2015 found that overall, people with a balanced outlook on life were more enthusiastic and passionate about their jobs and felt less hurried and rushed than others. They never felt too busy, nor did they feel overwhelmed by their schedule. If you feel pressed for time, there is a good chance that you do not enjoy what you do. Life might be like that at times, but if you start to feel overburdened, adding one additional, enjoyable activity to your day, something that keeps you engaged and entertained, might help.

Have you ever noticed that when you're passionate about something, it seems like you have more time for it? Scientists have looked into this and found that when employees don't have passion for their jobs, they feel like their goals conflict with each other, which can make it hard to balance work and family time. For example, someone who wants to succeed at work might have a hard time making it home for dinner with their family. But when people are passionate about their work, they see their work and personal life as complementary. They believe that spending time with family and doing other things they enjoy actually gives them more energy and motivation to do well at work. So when we're short on time, it's not just about doing tasks that are fun. It's also important to find tasks that align with our values and goals. If our goals conflict with each other, we're more likely to feel like we don't have enough time in our lives.

While we may voluntarily choose some of our responsibilities, others are largely the result of our society or culture. When we don't choose our responsibilities, we start to feel that we are not living up to society's standards. Remember, a lot of things we do in our lives are done not because we *want* to do them but because we *must* do them. This is where the principle of "Hll Yeah," or "N.O. capital N, capital O" comes in handy. If you are experiencing inner conflict about doing something, perhaps you're better off not doing it at all. There is a chance the task was not something you wanted to do but something that was imposed on you by social norms, co-workers, friends or family and culture.

The Beast Mode lifestyle is all about rising above your perceptions and believing you have sole control over time. You're not going to be able to develop the attitude and mindset that you dictate your own time in a day. We will talk more about developing habits that give you time in the following sections of this chapter.

The psychology behind the idea that we don't have enough time is complicated, but it is the primary reason that we cannot find time for what is important and what is valuable. In addition to our minds, there are many other objective reasons that squeeze our schedules and narrow down our leisure. However, with the right mindset, it is possible to deal with all of them. Here are some worth mentioning:

- Being a single parent
- Being a new parent
- Bad habit of waking up late
- Having to work two jobs at once
- Having to support a large family alone

These are all reasons you might have a tight schedule and find it increasingly difficult to manage your time yourself. However, adopting the Beast Mode attitude means you rise above all complications and troubles and live to your full potential. Beast Mode is about developing the mindset and harnessing the habits to help you live the life of your dreams, despite setbacks.

BEAST MODE LIFESTYLE TO FREE UP MORE TIME

Time management is the skill of planning and arranging so that you can free up time to be productive and reach your desired objectives. It involves taking responsibility for your own life and actively choosing how you spend your time. As we discussed in the psychology of time in the previous section, the majority of complaints regarding a lack of time start with ourselves. We are guilty of mismanaging our own time, whether we accept it or not.

Before getting into some of the practical steps you can take to improve your time management skills, let's talk about how you can shift your mindset for the better.

The first and primary tip of time management is understanding that you control your own time. Time is priceless and also very limited. So, it is important you deliberately choose to do things that you really want to do. Develop the mindset of rising above society's expectations and focus on things that you believe in.

"Run your day—stop letting the day run you." – Jim Rohn

You need to internalize that you are in the driving seat of your life. Otherwise, all other productivity tips for managing time will be worthless.

You're probably going to argue that there are some things in life that we can't control, like fixed schedules or obligations. But have you ever thought about changing the way you approach the free time you do have? Instead of fixating on the few activities that take up most of your time, what if you looked at other ways to fit in the things you really want to do? By doing this, you could take control of your schedule and make the most of the time you have available. It's time to shift your perspective and stop letting external factors dictate your free time.

Here are some strategies you can employ to take back control of your time and be proactive in how you use it:

- **Prioritize:** It's easy to involve yourself in any task that comes your way, and you find yourself rushing to complete each item as it appears, regardless of its importance. But this is a recipe for losing control. Instead, use a priority matrix to organize your tasks by urgency.

	Urgent	Not Urgent
Important	#1 Do	#3 Plan
Not Important	#2 Delegate	#4 Delete

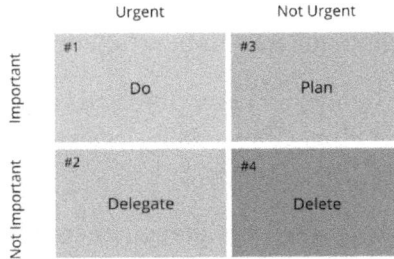

- Always look to complete your most urgent tasks first; these are the activities that require you to take instant action and may include deadlines, taking your child to school, etc. Therefore, not completing these tasks can result in severe consequences.

- **Filter out unnecessary info:** It's common for men to get sidetracked by unnecessary information, which can lead to a significant waste of time. With the constant barrage of information we face daily, it's easy to lose focus and waste valuable time on trivial matters. For instance, we recently witnessed a businessman spending an hour watching "tech reels" despite not being a tech enthusiast. As a result, he probably complained about being busy at the end of the day without realizing that he had wasted an hour on something unimportant. To truly unleash your productivity and achieve your goals using the Beast Mode, it's important to focus on the things that matter most to you. By filtering out unnecessary distractions and focusing on useful information, you can increase your chances of success and accomplish what you need to do.

- **Say no:** Saying no is a big part of valuing things that are important to you instead of giving in to peer pressure. Repeating this mantra to yourself will empower you to stand behind your decisions and prioritize your own needs. It's impossible to realize how much free time you will buy using a simple "NO." Most men struggle to concentrate on their own objectives and time since they are too easily distracted by others and feel bad for declining invitations. If you let other people interrupt you and make their issues your own, even if you are extremely driven and organized, you will continue to waste important time. Stick to your goals and use the power of no to stay on track.

Additionally, you could:

- ensure you know exactly what outcome you want from the planned activity,
- use a daily planner
- use the Pomodoro Technique to break your work into thirty-minute chunks, or
- eliminate distractions

Time management is a skill that anyone can develop; it's not rocket science. However, you need to let go of preconceived notions and develop the Beast Mode mindset and attitude. It's easy to get distracted by constant interruptions and other issues that interfere with your daily plans, making it difficult to take control of your time. Nevertheless, time is a crucial resource that every man should prioritize.

Anybody who hasn't mastered time management has no chance of mastering life. Time is one of our most precious assets, and how we utilize it is completely up to us. It is a well known fact that a Millionaire and a beggar both have 24 hours in a day. The only difference between them is how they use their time.

CHAPTER 3

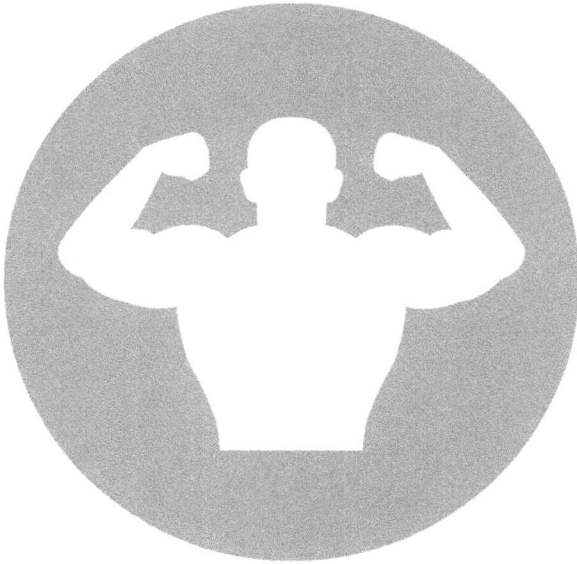

PHYSICAL
HEALTH

3

PHYSICAL HEALTH

A healthy lifestyle leads to a healthy mindset. How concerned are modern men with their physical health? Remote work, an unhealthy diet, and a lack of physical exercise have turned many men into couch potatoes. If given a choice between slacking on a couch or going for a run, very few men will pick the latter. We learned about the importance of exercise at a very early age, so why are men so apathetic about it? What are some of the main obstacles preventing men from exercising?

Our tendency to conserve energy and avoid physical exercise is an evolutionary response that was useful in the past when calories were scarce. However, as our lifestyle has become more sedentary, this response has become a bad habit that harms our health. To overcome this, we must shift our mindset and use our Beast Mode attitude to prioritize physical activity and take care of our bodies, even it if goes against our natural instinct to conserve energy.

In this chapter, we talk about how the Beast Mode mindset and attitude will help you create your ideal physique so you can develop and move toward your fitness goals.

. . .

REAL REASONS MEN AVOID EXERCISE

Automation, computerization, urbanization, and passive leisure all reduce men's physical activity levels. Today, we circle a parking lot for ten minutes to get a spot closer to the entrance. We wait to use the elevator to get to the first floor. We can order basically anything from anywhere with the touch of a button. This drastic shift from an active to a sedentary lifestyle has happened in a relatively short period and comes with multiple negative side effects. Our general lack of physical activity has created a culture of obesity as well as an increased incidence of diabetes, heart disease, cancer, and other disorders.

Studies reveal that more than 25 percent of people in America do not engage in any physical exercise AT ALL, and more than 60 percent of American adults do not meet the recommended levels of physical activity ("President's Council on Sports, Fitness & Nutrition," n.d.).

But we know all this, don't we? We know that a lack of physical exercise is harmful to our body, mind, and soul. Then why not exercise thirty minutes a day?

"It's Hard Work": Face it, exercising is not always fun and games. It's harder than most things you do in your day-to-day life. When you start exercising, everything starts to hurt. Your knees, your back, your chest, every muscle in your body. Most often, people make a mistake. They remain determined that they are going to exercise five times per week. They feel the burn, and after three days, their body starts giving up. Their motivation, commitment, and resolution to exercise and get fit are done and dusted before the journey has even begun. We will talk about how the Beast Mode mindset will help you leave this behind later in this chapter.

"I don't have the time": One of the easiest excuses to make. Time is relative. Most often, we use this excuse when we believe we have other important things to do in our lives. We do not prioritize exercise. So many men make this same excuse. These are the same men who spend hours and hours scrolling through social media wasting their time doing nothing productive.

Thirty minutes is only two percent of your day. Can you dedicate two percent of your time to your physical health so that you can live a healthier and happier life afterward? You may claim that exercise just does not fit into your hectic schedule, whether it's because of your job, family, kids, or a mix of these. However, the reality is: you *do* have the ability to manage time; you just don't want to or you haven't made your health a priority yet.

"It's intimidating": Many men who haven't worked out before might find going to the gym intimidating. Especially when it feels like it serves as the epicenter of emasculation. However, there is another factor at play that's hard to describe yet important to understand.

Have you heard of Schrodinger's cat? It's a thought experiment where a cat is put in a box with a fifty-fifty chance of eating poisoned food and dying. Until the box is opened, the cat could still be alive. But if you open the box and the cat is dead, you're essentially responsible for its death. This phenomenon is known as the observer's phenomenon—it means that observations determine result.

For a man, going to the gym can feel like Schrodinger's cat. As long as he doesn't see himself fail to bench press the forty-five-pound bar, he still believes he's strong. So, in a way, there is no way to tell for sure if he's weak unless he goes to the gym. While this might sound like a masculinity myth, there are many men who think this way and as a result, avoid the gym altogether.

"It's not working": When we live in such an instantly gratifying reality, its easy to see why more and more men are becoming impatient. They want results, and they expect them fast. Men are looking to torch fat, build the physique of their dreams, and live up to the same body standards that Instagram fitness influencers or celebrities show online and in the media. These same influencers only add fuel to the fire when they advertise their courses promising to halve your weight in fourteen days.

These false promises, complemented by false reviews, create a notion in men's minds that they are incapable of exercising. So they give up altogether. We know it can be frustrating when you're not reaching your fitness goals as fast as you'd like to but it's important to remember that fitness and physical health cannot be hacked. It is a gradual process that's going to take time and effort.

"Where do I start": The internet is filled with fitness influencers who say they know what they're doing. Everyone has a different opinion. If you start searching for workout guidelines, you will get an array of advice. You can choose from programs such as high-intensity interval training (HIIT), Pump, RPM, CrossFit, Yoga, Pilates, Piloxy, Boxing, F45, or Orange Theory. Your friends, family, and concerned know-it-alls will advise you not to run, not to lift, to be cautious of this and cautious of that, and so on. The best thing to do is to talk with your fitness trainer and not pay heed to what you hear from other people who don't have the results you seek.

"I don't feel motivated": Motivation is perhaps the number one reason why people fail to begin an exercise routine. Getting up and out every day to work out for thirty minutes requires mental effort. Many start their workout regimens just to give up. Some become disheartened when they do not see improvements in their bodies quickly enough. Some just don't enjoy themselves. Whatever the reason might be, holding on to motivation is one of the hardest things to do when trying to exercise regularly. Once you lose motivation, it becomes increasingly more difficult to get back on track the next time. It is said that motivation is like a hot shower, its nice and warm whilst you are in it but the minute you step out, its freezing cold again! You need to find reasons to act whether you 'feel' like it or not. We will discuss the fundamentals of motivation in greater depth in the second book of this series.

"I can't afford it": So many people get ahead of themselves. They make a resolution on December 31 and buy all the expensive gear and membership the next day. They work out for seven days and quit. The result? All that money goes to waste. When you ask them to go work out the next time, they come up with the excuse that they cannot afford it.

Exercising doesn't need to be expensive; you don't necessarily need to join a gym and pay its monthly or yearly subscription fees. You can exercise from anywhere at any time, and we'll discuss all the ways you can do this later in this chapter.

In reality, there are very few valid reasons for not exercising. The reason we make excuses is that we have a subconscious need to maintain our sense of self-worth. We use excuses as a defense mechanism to protect our sense of self against the typical challenges of daily life. We come up with silly excuses instead of admitting that we simply do not want to exercise. However, the Beast Mode mindset teaches us to reject these excuses and overcome the obstacles that prevent us from achieving our goals. Let's use the Beast Mode mindset to counteract our excuses and take control of our physical health.

GOODBYE EXCUSES. HELLO RESULTS

To improve our quality of life, we must adopt the Beast Mode mindset and overcome the obstacles that prevent us from achieving our health goals, which often remain unfulfilled due to procrastination. We try to look for shortcuts to earning good health, but the problem is, there aren't any. While it's OK to be flexible with your fitness objectives, making good habits like exercise a regular part of your life will majorly influence your overall health and well-being.

Boosting your motivation to work out can be difficult as you are essentially trying to persuade your own mind to do something it may not want to do. Conventional methods of thinking may not have been effective for you, but there are other ways to increase motivation.

Here are some tips to help you build the motivation you need to work out:

Reward yourself: Your brain is wired for instant gratification. It craves rewards and wants everything as soon as possible. In his book *The Power of Habit*, Charles Duhig discusses how you can make anything more palatable by giving yourself instant rewards.

For instance, you could reward yourself by watching an episode of your favorite series every time you work out for thirty minutes. Duhig also talks about creating a "habit loop," which includes: a signal to start whatever it is you need to do (something like placing your running shoes next to your bed), the routine (like finishing thirty minutes of a workout), and finally, the reward (watching an episode on Netflix). The reason an extrinsic reward is so potent is that your brain will connect it to the habit, making it more likely that the routine will stick.

The chemicals known as endorphins are responsible for giving you that satisfying "I feel great" sensation after a tough workout. As the brain begins to associate these chemicals with the physical exertion and perspiration of exercise, the drive to work out becomes more ingrained. Once you recognize that the workout in and of itself is the ultimate gratification, the allure of a Netflix episode will no longer hold sway over you.

Remap positive thinking: There are lots of devotees to positive thinking who talk about how visualizing has motivated them toward healthy habits. Visualization means imagining yourself in the circumstances you want to be in. Athletes often imagine themselves winning a race, scoring a goal, winning a fight, or becoming champions in their sport in order to boost their motivation. However, according to Gabriele Oettingen, the author of *Rethinking Positive Thinking: Inside the New Science of Motivation*, such a formula of positive visualization is only half complete.

After deciding what you truly want and visualizing the outcome, you need to figure out what's stopping you from getting it. The author calls this process "mental contrasting." In one study of fifty-one female students who claimed they wanted to eat less junk food, researchers asked each to envision the advantages of doing so. The people who were most effective at keeping to their goal were those who recognized what made it harder for them to eat healthily and devised a strategy to eat fruit when cravings struck. (Oettingen, 2009)

Utilize this mental principle. Feeling too worn out to exercise after work? Rather than coming up with the excuse of "being too tired," switch to morning or lunchtime workouts or head directly to the gym after work to overcome the hurdle.

Find your tribe: We believe our health to be our own. We feel as though it is something no one can help us with. But we are wrong. Although being responsible for yourself is great, being alone on a journey can be demotivating. Instead of trying to work things out all alone, a strong, encouraging community will ultimately keep us going long-term.

Has a friend ever complimented you and turned your whole day around when you were miserable? The same can happen with working out. Having a like-minded group of people beside you can also make exercising more enjoyable. Regardless of your current level of fitness or your objectives, having fun will motivate you. Fitness is important, but it doesn't have to be so serious. A supportive community may help you remember that although working toward your fitness objectives is essential, so are having fun and laughing; you don't have to choose just one.

Motivation is crucial to establishing fitness objectives, staying dedicated, and persevering in the face of difficulty. By using the principles we mentioned, you can maintain your motivation for longer and achieve the physical health you desire.

SECRETS TO CONSISTENT WORKOUTS

Starting a workout routine is easy; maintaining the routine is more challenging. You will come across many obstacles that make it difficult to stay committed to your health goals. While setting fitness goals are great, it will take way more than planning to be successful. Consistency is tough, but it is also super powerful.

You only need to improve by 1 percent each day to improve. Then, over the year, this 1 percent will compound and grow and, before you know it, you will have met your goals. Consistency converts a routine into a habit and a habit into a lifestyle. When you consistently work out, you start incorporating it into your life. Sooner or later, you will be so accustomed to it that you won't have to put in any extra effort to see it through.

Here are some ways you can develop consistency with your workouts:

Start small: You don't have to run a marathon on your first day. To make it easier to establish a consistent exercise routine, it's recommended to start small. Instead of jumping into a rigorous workout schedule right away, consider doing ten-minute workouts. This approach has two benefits:

1. It helps you avoid muscle pain and burnout in the first few days, making it easier to keep the ball rolling and make exercise part of your daily routine.
2. Everyone has a spare five or ten minutes, so it's a quick and easy way to overcome any excuses for not exercising.

Within these ten-minute workouts, you could do pushups as you watch television, squats while you fold clothes, or walk around your neighborhood. Over time, you will find more time and motivation to continue for five more minutes, then five more, and so on. We dive deeper into physical health and fitness in the second book of the Beast Mode series, which goes into greater detail about exercise and explores movement patterns at a more advanced level. If you'd like to learn more about exercise, we'd highly recommend you keep an eye out for it.

Break down your goals: Establishing specific objectives is a fantastic way to get back in the game, and research has shown that doing so really encourages behavior change with regard to nutrition and exercise (Shilts, 2004). However, it's important to establish the correct *type* of goals. An overly ambitious goal may be difficult to maintain. So, we advise you to develop SMART objectives.

S = Specific

M = Measurable

A = Achievable

R = Relevant

T = Time-bound

Your goals need to comply with all of the above. Only then will your objectives be realistic and manageable. You might feel this is counterintuitive since everyone talks about aiming "sky high," but we have a story to help you understand this strategy and its importance.

You are determined to reduce 15 kilos of body weight within three months, so you create a fitness regimen. The default setting on your step counter is ten thousand steps per day. While it seems possible, you continuously fall short; on most days, you only reach eight thousand. You set an unattainable objective, and you feel awful about yourself.

The solution is simple: make your goal feasible by starting small. You want to teach your brain to believe you can succeed. If you lower your target to eight thousand steps, you will regularly achieve this, and it will give you strength, confidence, and capability. Once you have gained confidence in your abilities to achieve the daily target, you can gradually up your step count until it reaches twelve thousand steps each day. It may take six weeks, but because of the immediate pleasure you get from meeting your target, you realize that you have reached your goal or even exceeded it. Starting small inspires you to do better and keep going.

Start with achievable goals and work your way up. The more victories you have along the way, the more motivated you will be.

Go with the flow—be flexible: Some men habitually go to the gym every morning at 6 a.m. before work. However, if they wake up ten minutes late, they will simply avoid going to the gym altogether. Why is this? It's because they think they'll be late for work if they go to the gym in the morning instead, rather than realizing they could place the time for exercise elsewhere in their schedules. Just because you miss your 6 a.m. "slot," it doesn't mean you can't do anything at 6 p.m.

We need to adopt a "go with the flow" mentality. You cannot be too strict and regimented. Our lives are spontaneous, and they don't always go to plan. So, you always need to have a plan B, C, and D to fall back on when things don't go as you imagined. If you wake up late in the morning, you can always plan to work out after work.

Many of us have strict ideas about what constitutes exercise, but there are innumerable ways to move throughout the day if you can't make it to the gym. You need to become more adaptable in how you include exercise throughout your day. If you can't go to the gym to work out, you can always:

- run in the park for thirty minutes,
- do pushups, squats and crunches,
- walk up and down the stairs for fifteen minutes, or
- jump rope for 20 minutes.

There is a whole load of things you can do to go with the flow. Don't avoid exercise all together just because you missed the slot in your schedule.

Give up the "all or nothing" mindset: So many people begin their fitness regimen with great enthusiasm, but when they're derailed even once, they completely fall off the wagon.

You may say things like:

"I'm going to start losing weight in January..."

"I'm going to start working out after the holidays..."

These examples are instances of the "all or nothing" attitude, and they can be self-destructive. When we bear this mindset, we crave perfection to succeed, leading to unrealistic expectations and a fear of failure that holds us back from trying out new things.

We've all been there, but it's important we reframe our thoughts about health. Instead of striving for perfection, aim for progress. Jog around the neighborhood when you don't have time for a full workout; while it's not perfect, it'll keep your workout streak intact. Life is full of uncertainty, and you can never plan for all outcomes. It's better if you learn to adapt and continue making progress.

Keeping these points in mind will help you consistently work out, but before that, you need to make a start. Not tomorrow, not next Sunday, but today. If you have no idea how to exercise, we will add some regimens you can try at the end of this chapter. However, if you want to try out more advanced workout programs, check out the second book in this series, where we delve deeper into improving men's fitness, nutrition, and well-being.

Remember, the Beast Mode mindset and attitude embraces action more than motivation. If you have to wait for motivation to come to you, you'll be waiting a long time. Don't wait; take action NOW!

MONEY SAVING FITNESS HACKS

A common excuse is, "I can't afford it." Who said you need a credit-draining gym membership or expensive equipment in the first place? Physical exercise is not expensive, but not making it a priority can prove costly.

The internet and all its fitness influencers tell you to buy the latest and greatest gadgets in order to do the most effective exercise. It can be depressing and repelling, particularly if you are unable to fit it all into your budget. Committing to working out regularly is challenging enough as it is; adding financial stress can make it seem unattainable.

Taking care of your health does not have to be expensive, despite what the media says. In fact, physical exercise does not have to cost any money at all. You don't have to let your financial situation prevent you from achieving your fitness goals. The only thing you really need is a strong will.

Here are some strategies to help you work out, basically for free:

Workout at home: Your home might not have sophisticated machines and trainers to help you work out, but it's a great place to start when you're a newbie. You don't need to spend money on a gym membership immediately. Give yourself time to work out at home and get used to the routine first.

Some home workout resources include:

- **Exercise videos:** There are hundreds of thousands of exercise videos available for all ages and fitness levels on YouTube. From yoga and Pilates to HIIT and dance workouts, YouTube offers a diverse range of options for people to stay active and healthy. Take time to explore the platform and find the workouts best for you.
- **Outdoor workouts:** You can always take a brisk walk or jog around your neighborhood or nearby park. All you need is a good pair of shoes. You can also use outdoor playground equipment to perform pull-ups, push-ups, and other bodyweight exercises. Monkey bars can be used for hanging and swinging exercises, while park benches can be used for step-ups, triceps dips, chest presses, box jumps, and other exercises. Find hills or stairs to incorporate sprinting or incline workouts into your routine.
- **Home appliances:** Now, this might sound silly. But this is what the whole Beast Mode mindset is all about. Use what you have at home as pieces of gym equipment; for example, use full milk or water bottles as weights. Be

resourceful and turn your chores into an opportunity for physical activity.

Use inexpensive fitness gear: Having fancy gym equipment is nice, but it doesn't guarantee you will have a great workout. Instead, try smaller, more affordable equipment, such as:

- **Resistance Bands.** These are cheap and can be easily stored in a drawer. Resistance bands are very handy for working on every muscle in the body.
- **Kettlebells.** These are versatile and can provide a full-body workout. They can be used for a wide range of exercises and movements, such as swings, snatches, and goblet squats.
- **Jump ropes.** These are used by highly-trained elite boxers and professional fighters for conditioning and endurance. Jump ropes offer a versatile and affordable cardio exercise that can be done anywhere and can be tailored to your fitness level.

Use what you already have: Most of us already have some fitness gear at home that we've just never used. If you don't want to use household items or purchase any equipment, check your garage or basement for any sports items you might have bought and forgotten about. If you discover anything in decent condition, see if you can utilize it for your exercises. These items might include:

- Baseballs, footballs, and basketballs
- Tennis rackets
- Bicycles
- Frisbees
- Paddleball games
- Mini trampolines
- Mini steppers
- Boxing gloves or pads

You're the only thing standing in your way when it comes to exercising. You don't need expensive gear; you don't need a gym membership; you don't need extra motivation; you don't need extra time. All you need is the determination to take care of your health and the willpower to see it through.

BEYOND AVERAGE WORKOUTS TO GET YOU ON TRACK

Are you ready to unleash your inner beast? Hearing "Beast Mode" might conjure up images of big muscles and six-pack abs, but it's really all about mentality and attitude. Ordinary men are easily derailed from their fitness objectives, finding excuses and procrastinating instead of taking action. But with the right mindset, you can become a true beast and achieve your fitness goals. Remember, progress may not happen overnight, but with determination, you can achieve better health.

Now you're motivated, it's important to come up with a plan of action, particularly if you're unused to regular exercise or don't know how to form a routine to help you meet your objectives. Consider starting by focusing on cardio or strength.

Cardio: Cardio increases your aerobic endurance. Depending on your current fitness level, a challenging cardio exercise can be as simple as a brisk walk. The idea is to increase your heart rate and make you breathe harder to circulate more oxygen into your muscles. This is true of all cardio exercises, including cycling, swimming, running, etc. Cardio workouts not only help increase your endurance but also enhance your body's composition.

Start with a low to moderate intensity. If you choose jogging, walk for a few minutes, run for a few minutes, and repeat for at least ten minutes in the beginning. No matter how you choose to exercise, your cardio should initially be limited to ten to fifteen minutes. Increase your workout's length and intensity gradually to prevent injury.

Strength: There are several techniques for building muscular strength and endurance. You can use dumbbells, sandbags, resistance bands, barbells, and so on, and you can work out either at the gym or at home. Strength exercises incorporating lighter weights and more repetitions will increase your muscular endurance, whereas heavier weights and fewer reps will increase your muscles' strength and size. Here is a routine designed by fitness instructor Sayer that you can follow at home:

- 25 jumping jacks
- 15 bodyweight squats
- 20–30 second plank
- Walking lunges—10 per side
- 10 push-ups (on knees if you need to)
- 30 seconds running in place with high knees
- 15 glute bridges
- 30 seconds Russian twist
- 10 lateral lunges per side
- 15 Superman back extensions
- 15 bent-knee triceps dips off the edge of a bench or chair (straighten your legs if they are too easy)
- Repeat all steps once more

(Sayer, 2022)

Here is another regimen you can try if you have access to gym equipment:

- 30 seconds mountain climbers
- 12 squats with dumbbells at shoulder height
- 10 reps of step-ups with overhead press per side
- 12 reps of chest press with dumbbells
- 12 deadlifts with a barbell or dumbbell
- 20 stability ball crunches
- 12 reps of biceps curls
- 12 reps per side of bent-over single-arm rows

- 12 dumbbell triceps extensions per side
- 30-second plank
- 12 reps of bent-over reverse fly with dumbbells
- Repeat all steps once more

(Sayer, 2022)

Now that you have a workout routine to get you started, begin as soon as you can, preferably right away. However, remember the following tips to make your exercises even more successful:

- Begin each exercise with a brief period of warm-up.
- Stretch both before and after exercise to increase your flexibility and reduce pain.
- Do not push yourself. Start slowly by alternating between rest days and activity days.
- If you experience discomfort or extreme weariness during any workout, stop right away.
- Switch up your workouts and try new things to stay interested and motivated.
- Consume enough water before, during, and after exercise.

Unleashing your Beast Mode requires you to be at your physical and mental best, and physical exercise is a way to achieve both. Exercising can help improve every aspect of your life, such as your mental health, work stress, relationship issues, and low self-esteem. It's not about showing off your physique to get attention; it's about you and your journey to becoming the best you can be. It is certainly a long and difficult process, but the path to being physically and mentally healthy has no shortcut.

It is about grit, determination, and willpower.

CHAPTER 4

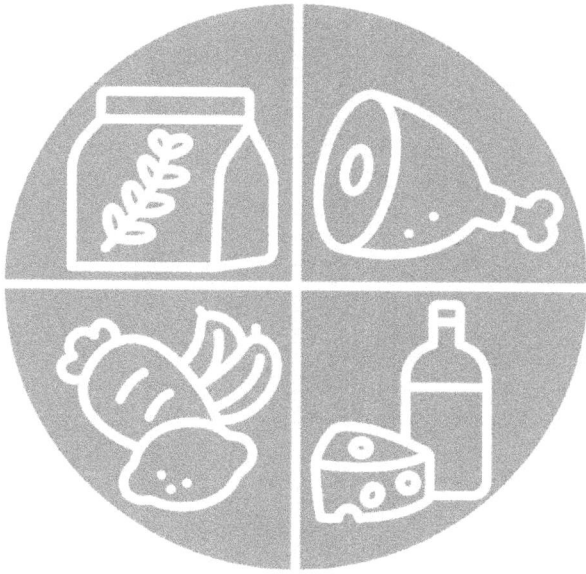

FOOD & NUTRITION

4

FOOD & NUTRITION

I t's essential to take care of both fitness and nutrition to achieve good physical health. Unfortunately, many men tend to ignore the food they consume, which leads to a higher incidence of chronic diseases like diabetes mellitus, hypertension, and stroke. Therefore, it's important to examine the relationship between men's diets and these conditions, as a healthy diet can help prevent them. Historically, women have been responsible for purchasing, preparing, and providing food, and this has led to men being less aware of the health benefits of certain foods. However, it's vital to note that even if men had this knowledge, many still show a general disinterest in taking care of their bodies. This may be due to societal expectations that praise men who eat more or indulge in unhealthy food.

OVERCOMING BARRIERS TO NUTRITIONAL EATING

There is no shortage of excuses for not maintaining a healthy diet. Even though the science behind having a healthy life is extremely straightforward and most men do want to eat better to lose weight and build more muscle, applying it is challenging. That's why attitude is everything. If you make nutritious, healthy meals a priority, you will make time to shop for groceries and prepare healthy meals in your daily life. Here are some of men's most common struggles regarding eating healthily:

"I'm not sure where to start": Trying to maintain a healthy diet can seem like a massive deal when you are just starting out; people get bogged down by just the thought of transitioning to a perfect diet. However, no one is born knowing everything, so you can always learn. You don't need to make night and day changes to your diet; even the tiniest adjustments will be helpful once you learn what you need to alter.

Just START. You don't need specialized training to eat healthily. You don't need to consult a dietitian or read long books to learn all there is to know about it. Start with the very basics. Minimise intake of processed food and start eating more wholefoods including proteins, vegetables, fruits, nuts and seeds. We will talk more about diets in the coming sections of the chapter.

"It's overwhelming": You might find it overwhelming to exercise regularly and follow a balanced diet. You might think you are being too hard on yourself. Men often don't appreciate the benefits of doing so and instead think about all the hard work they'd have to do to maintain their lifestyle. So, they give up after a week.

What you can do instead is start small and make one good health choice each day. For instance, plan to limit dine-outs to only twice a month. Gradually you can add healthier food choices to your daily schedule. You can always start small and work your way up.

"I have to lose so much weight; it is impossible": This is a self-defeating statement. There are so many people who see how far they have to climb to reach their goals and give up before even starting. Your defeat usually stems from having limiting beliefs, which are easy to have and difficult to change. However, it isn't impossible, and building a growth mindset will help you not only with your health goals, but with all other aspects of your life, too.

That's why reframing your mindset is important. Rather than concentrating on a goal that seems far off, think about making modest adjustments that will get you closer to a healthier version of yourself. Honor development above perfection.

"I'm too old for a balanced diet now": No, you are not. There is no age or time to start taking care of your health. Even if you're in your fifties and have been diagnosed with major ailments, the human body is intended to adapt. Your body is constantly prepared to improve its health, no matter your age and no matter the disease.

"My schedule is too busy right now": We discussed this in the previous chapter, too. A sad truth about life is that it is always going to be hectic. No matter what you do and what you achieve, life is never going to give you time off. Therefore, you have to make time for yourself; you can't wait for life to cut you some slack.

So don't put off taking control of your health until some hypothetical, perfect future moment. You will never be able to achieve the fitness you want by waiting. The problem with most men is that they don't make health a big priority; they consider it a luxury that they do not necessarily need to give in to until a major ailment such as a stroke, diabetes or heart attack forces them to.

"I deserve a treat": Justifying a junk food binge as a reward for your hard work shouldn't be confused with emotional eating, which is when you turn to food in times of stress. Yes, you do deserve a treat every now and then; however, you don't deserve an unhealthy body. Allow yourself treats but make sure you don't go overboard. There are lots of healthy alternatives to choose from.

"It's just genetics": It's so easy to blame genetics and not take responsibility for your physical health. After all, there's no use beginning a diet or fitness regimen if you're genetically predisposed to having a huge bottom or muffin top. I'm not against science; your genes *do* influence your body type and how readily fat is deposited in your body. However, you are still able to influence your body too.

In fact, evidence shows that the benefits of "fat genes" are outweighed by regular exercise ("Realbuzz," n.d.). So, you can still fight your genes with a healthy diet and activity plan, regardless of whether your family has instilled harmful eating habits in you at a young age or you are genetically predisposed to having an unhealthy body.

"Diets don't work for me": Weak men say anything to avoid a healthy diet, and this is just another one of those excuses. Do you really think you can have good health with that attitude? These people will say they "feel weak" when they follow a diet, they "lack the self-discipline" to stay with one, or they have never seen any noticeable effects.

However, as we have said many times in this book, the key to a healthy life is not great strategies and principles; it is all about mentality and attitude. If you are one of these men coming up with such excuses, perhaps your perception of and approach to your eating pattern needs to be re-assessed. You can't expect trying every fad diet that pops up in your newsfeed to give you long-lasting benefits or make you feel great about your health. Instead, abandon fad diets and switch to a practical, healthy eating strategy, making sure to give it a proper go before judging its efficacy.

"My metabolism is kinda slow": Some people use this as an excuse without knowing anything about metabolism. They believe that their metabolism is in between them and their health. But if you really have a sluggish metabolism, you need to follow healthy diets that speed it up. Exercise helps too.

"It's expensive": Many assert they cannot afford to eat healthier. However, in our opinion, healthy eating is much more budget-friendly than splurging on junk food. Buying an apple instead of a chocolate bar saves you money. Instead of dining out, buying raw chicken and fish in bulk and choosing whole or unsweetened, unsalted frozen food is going to save you money. We will talk more about saving money in the next chapter.

Start by cutting down on your portion sizes and replace your unhealthy snacks with fresh fruits or vegetables. Healthy food is just another excuse that you are coming up with in order to avoid it. If you look around, healthy foods are way cheaper than junk foods. What you don't pay for now by eating processed foods, you will in the long run with medical expenses and medication to counteract the effects of your poor food choices.

"Michael is eating it, and he's still skinny, so I can eat it too": The first wrong aspect of this statement is that no matter how skinny a person is, it doesn't guarantee he's healthy. Remember that we are not aware of others' diets. You don't know if your friend is eating unhealthy food ten times a day or if this is a once-in-a-year treat. You also have no idea how much he exercises. But what you need to know most is that you are not Michael.

It is you who is responsible for your own health and not Michael. You need to prioritize it without being influenced by the habits of others.

"Healthy food tastes bad": Another common excuse that could not be farther from the truth. Healthy does not mean bland. We could list a ton of tasty foods that are healthy (and we will do so later). While I appreciate that you may be inclined to make your favorite food sometimes, your priority should be to find and cook recipes that meet the criteria of both health and taste.

"One bite won't hurt": This is true. However, it's important to be mindful about what you're eating. While you don't need to cut any certain foods out entirely—it's important to allow yourself a treat! Be careful that a bag of potato chips doesn't turn into two. You don't want your well-intentioned snack to turn into a binge. As well as being unhealthy, it will mean you're more likely to think, *I've already blown it today; I'll start my diet tomorrow.* Remember: consume everything in moderation.

Most men make the excuses we've noted here. It's normal and natural. However, you want to be better than these excuses—that's why you've picked up this book. You want to tackle your mindset, limiting beliefs, and lack of knowledge to unlock your Beast Mode and become the best version of yourself. If you have these beliefs, it's probably that you're currently in your comfort zone and are subconsciously afraid of leaving it. That's okay; more men are! But growth happens outside the comfort zone, and this book is here to empower you to leave it.

BEAST MODE LIFESTYLE TO FUEL THE BEAST WITHIN

Eating is not difficult. Making wise food choices, however, is challenging. We are not going to make you follow a strict diet; that's not what this book is about. However, you shouldn't settle for mediocre choices that leave you sluggish and hungry. Nutrition fuels your inner beast and unleashes your potential. Choose nutrient-dense foods that nourish your body and energize your spirit. Remember, every meal is an opportunity to take one step closer to greatness. So, grab that knife and fork, and let's learn how to feast like a champion!

Instead of a diet mentality, what you need is a better way of thinking about how you view nutrition and food. When people make you follow a diet, you are less concerned with following your intuition and more concerned with following guidelines. This makes eating healthy more overwhelming. The dieting attitude includes:

- Putting a ban on some foods or entire food groups
- Avoiding food that you love eating
- Having set goals about reaching a number on the scales rather than encouraging overall health and well-being
- Spending on medications and supplements

We want to emphasize that we're not pushing you to diet. Instead, let's take a look at some things you can do to change your mindset about food and nutrition.

Understanding the *why*: A disciplined man doesn't take care of his health just because someone else is. The *why* is important. While it's unlikely you will follow through on anything if someone forces you to, if you are aware of the rewards and motivations to do something, it will be much simpler to maintain long-term habits and pick them up again when you fall off-track. This is why you need to consider your motivations for eating healthy carefully. Do you want abs? Do you want more energy? Do you want to enhance your overall health? There is no correct answer to this, but you do need to find your "reason why" yourself.

We advise you to consider "whys" that will stand the test of time. The more justifications you can discover for improving your lifestyle, the better.

Change your relationship with food: Building a better relationship with food is a crucial step toward healthy eating. Food should be both for sustenance and enjoyment. While most of the food you consume should be nutritional, it's also okay to enjoy the foods you love (even if they're a little unhealthy), as this will help you sustain your healthy eating patterns for longer. It's important to understand that food is neither good nor evil. It's not awful of you to indulge in your favorite food, whether that's chocolates, burgers and fries, pizzas, donuts, or anything else. Your health won't be ruined by it. No single meal is "fattening" or unhealthy until you consume it in excess over a period of time. This is when you'll gain unwanted weight.

People all too often try to ban a certain type of food from their diet altogether. Doing this will only make you crave it more. We presume that "healthy eating" means eating only salad, and we place labels on foods that are perfectly fine to consume in moderation. Instead of labeling food as good or bad, you must understand that you don't need to cut all your most-loved snacks out and be miserable for the sake of "healthy eating." You can still enjoy your favorite foods while managing your weight and overall health.

Don't compare your process with anyone: We know how hard it is to keep from comparing your body, weight, and physique with others. In our heads, we constantly ask ourselves:

- Am I eating more than them?
- Am I eating less than them?
- Would that person do this?
- Why can *he* do it, and I can't?

It's important to evaluate whether your standards for "healthy eating" are reasonable and based on accurate information, rather than comparing yourself to those with unhealthy habits. If you find yourself feeling doubtful despite introspections, it's best to avoid comparison altogether, and steer clear of conversations or social media promoting unhealthy eating patterns. Remember that the path to a healthy lifestyle is not a competition, and everyone has their own timeline. While it's natural to feel jealous of someone who has made significant improvements, there's no need to rush yourself.

Men with the Beast Mode mindset and attitude are proud of who they are. They do not compare themselves with others. They do not compare their process, either. Don't compare your success to others if you know you're doing what feels best for you and have a diet tailored to yourself. If you feel tempted to compare yourself, remember; everyone is unique.

Healthy eating is not hard work; it's self-care: We think healthy eating is something we must actively put effort into. We look at junk food as a reward and vegetables as punishment. Instead, we need to start considering nutrition a part of self-care. Do not associate reward and punishment with food and nutrition.

You need to reframe your mindset to develop better eating habits. We tend to force ourselves to eat healthily, but this results in increased cravings, challenges, and frustration. No more! Don't start eating healthy because you *have* to. Start eating healthy because you *want* to. Fueling your body with good food and nutrition will have positive impacts on your mind and body. In contrast, consuming too much processed foods will make you lethargic, grumpy, and diabetes prone. Change your mindset and say, "I choose not to eat this food because the way it makes me feel is not worth it."

The attitude shift from "I can't" to "I don't want to" is subtle but powerful. This simple mindset shift can make a whole lot of difference in sticking to healthy foods and avoiding unhealthy ones. It gives you more control to meet your goals rather than feeling like you're following someone else's rules.

Be mindful of what you're eating: The Beast Mode mindset emphasizes the importance of mindfulness. Your rational mind is more capable and disciplined than your subconscious brain, which tends to nag you to indulge in unhealthy behaviors. When faced with tempting situations like fast food shops, it's essential to connect with your conscious mind to make an appropriate decision. Pausing and considering whether or not to eat the food is crucial for reaching your maximum potential as a person.

According to the Center for Mindful Eating, connecting with your conscious mind helps you become more aware of your behaviors, thoughts, emotions, and motives and gain insight into the causes of your unhealthy behaviors. By practicing mindfulness, you can make healthier choices and stay true to your goals.

Don't connect your emotions to food: Food isn't the way to manage your emotions. So many people eat when they're sad, angry, or tired rather than finding a healthy outlet. It's important that you gain the self-awareness to realize when you're *actually* hungry and distinguish this from when you're eating to "fill the void" so to speak.

Remember:

- If you are sleepy, get some rest.
- If you are upset, find someone to share your feelings with.
- If you are angry, try and figure out what's setting you off.

Think one day at a time: The path to a healthy lifestyle is tough and long. Although it's important to know your objectives and long-term goal, if you're bogged down by how difficult it will be to get there, it can be detrimental.

Therefore, you should keep your mind on the present. Focus on one meal, one trip to the store, and one day at a time. Don't stop to consider how many more meals it will take to reach your fitness goal, celebrate the success of each healthy meal instead.

SIMPLIFIED NUTRITION FOR THE MODERN MAN

According to research by the Center for Disease Control and Prevention, men consume roughly 2,618 calories per day, of which 15 percent are from protein, 35 percent are from fat, and 50 percent are from carbs (Weber, 2010). The typical American man's caloric consumption has increased by five hundred calories daily over the last thirty years, with roughly 80 percent of those calories coming from carbs. The average American only consumes half the recommended amounts of fruits and vegetables, meaning the majority of these extra calories are made up of sugars and starches, commonly known as "simple" carbohydrates.

This is unsurprising. Our daily diets consist primarily of convenience foods such as potato chips, bagels, donuts, pastries, and so on. Simply put, the average American man's diet is nothing but a shortcut to obesity, diabetes, heart disease, and all the complications that come with these.

If you've gotten this far into the book, you understand that we want to give you the knowledge to make your own healthy choices. Therefore, we've put together a nutrition strategy meant to assist you in replacing empty-calorie foods with those that are more wholesome and satiating.

Eliminate added sugar: According to research from the University of California, fructose—a naturally occurring sugar that is now present in almost everything—can trick your brain into craving more food even when already satisfied (Weber, 2010). This happens because fructose mutes your response to leptin, the "enough is enough" hormone. Therefore, sweetened foods tend to make us overeat.

We have uncovered numerous reasons why men do not follow dietary guidelines; however, we haven't yet mentioned how over-complicated today's guidelines are. Look at this straightforward, four-word US dietary recommendation from the 1980s:

"Limit your intake of sugar."

Yes, that's it. No eating plan, no guides, no walkthroughs; just plain and simple. On the other hand, the current guideline states:

"Choose and prepare foods and beverages with little added sugars or caloric sweeteners, such as amounts suggested by the USDA Food Guide and the DASH [Dietary Approaches to Stop Hypertension] Eating Plan."

To follow this advice, you'd need to search for the USDA and DASH suggested amounts, and who knows when the information will be updated again for the hundredth time. Stick to the 1980s approach and cut down on how often you eat foods with added sugar. In this way, you will:

- eliminate most junk foods from your daily diet,
- reduce your calorie intake, and
- immediately improve your diet without calculating calories.

You will also feel better knowing that you're consuming sugar when YOU want to and not because some deceitful food manufacturer slipped it into your Caesar salad dressing.

Add quality proteins: Regardless of whether you're vegetarian or not, it's a misconception that most of your protein comes from animal products. Our biggest source of protein is soy. Shocked? We were, too. You might say, "This doesn't apply to me; I don't eat a lot of tofu." Maybe you don't, but you *do* consume a lot more soy than you realize.

Soy is included in foods that claim to be "rich in protein," such as cereals and energy bars. The issue is that since soy protein isn't a "complete" protein like the protein found in meat, dairy, and fish, it lacks some essential amino acids required by your body to develop and maintain muscle. Genistein and daidzein, two naturally occurring substances found in soy, mimic estrogen and work to balance testosterone, a crucial hormone for sustaining muscle mass.

So, what we are taking in as protein is not actually a quality protein. We not only need to consume quality protein, but we also need more of it. While the USDA advises 56 grams per day, most adult men would benefit from consuming more.

And, no. You shouldn't start sipping raw eggs.

A protein-rich diet rich has advantages beyond building muscle. Protein satisfies hunger and helps prevent many chronic diseases. A decent general guideline is to consume 1 gram of protein for every pound of your target body weight. (In other words, consume 175 grams of protein if you wish to weigh 175 pounds.) Focus on dairy, eggs, fish, poultry, and beef cuts with the term "loin" in the name, such as sirloin or tenderloin.

Trade starch for whole grains: The primary component in white rice, white bread, and pasta is starch. Starches are rapidly and readily absorbed by the body. Since they are simply extended chains of sugar molecules, eating too much starch will cause hunger. The simple solution? Eat fruits and veggies.

Most fresh produce is high in fiber, rich in vitamins and minerals, low in calories, and low in starch. While dietitians are skilled at coming up with long lists of food to avoid, they never give the simple—and most effective—advice to cut the starch and eat the produce.

A sensible target is limiting your intake of starch to three or four servings per day. One serving is equivalent to around one slice of bread, one cup of cereal, half a big potato, or 1 cup of cooked pasta or rice. If you consume less starch and avoid items with added sugars, you'll have better blood sugar control and less acute carb cravings—the cravings that lead you to seek out fast solutions to hunger and choose unhealthy options.

It will be far better to replace empty calories with fiber-rich vegetables and whole grains. That is because, unlike sugar and carbohydrates, fiber remains intact until it is almost at the end of your digestive tract. A good goal is to multiply your current consumption of fruits and vegetables by three. The minimum recommended serving size for a healthy diet is five.

You can break these servings down by using the Plate Method. Using this method, you should ensure that for breakfast, lunch, and dinner:

- a quarter of your plate is filled with protein, such as chicken, fish, beef, pork, tofu, or lentils,
- a quarter is filled with starchy carbs, such as potatoes, rice, or bread, and
- half is filled with non-starchy fibrous vegetables, such as leafy greens, broccoli, cauliflower, or eggplant.

Embrace natural fats: There is no doubt that fat is bad for you —but only one type of fat: man-made trans-saturated fats. All our life, we have been led to believe that any kind of fat is unhealthy, which is a complete myth. Health concerns regarding cholesterol and saturated fat are quite exaggerated.

As more studies are completed on fat consumption, it has become apparent that trans-fats are directly related to high cholesterol, heart disease, stroke, and diabetes. Nutritionists now advise us to embrace fat, especially the fat found in meat and dairy products, and to concentrate on consuming heart-healthy mono and polyunsaturated fats found in foods like almonds, olive oil, and avocados.

Consume healthy fats present in whole foods such as milk, cheese, meat, avocados, nuts, and olive oil. Fat adds taste to meals and makes you feel full, both of which help you avoid overeating. Stop tormenting yourself by eating low-fat or no-fat junk food; there's no need to when you could choose to eat healthy fat.

The problem with dieting and nutrition is that we overcomplicate it and overwhelm ourselves. Keep it simple. Don't waste time and energy selecting a specific diet. Instead, follow the tips above to set yourself up for the healthy lifestyle you've always wanted.

UNMASKING THE TRUTHS BEHIND HEALTHY EATING

Part of living a Beast Mode lifestyle is fueling yourself with wholesome nutritional food, but this won't be possible while businesses are funding misleading advertising and marketing anything as healthy. It's important that you can make your own informed choices about what you put into your body. Therefore, we're going to reveal the strategies food companies use so that you can protect yourself against them.

Here are some myths they are trying to preach:

"Beverages marketed as 'healthy' are actually healthy": From sweetened green tea to vitamin-enhanced waters, beverage companies are marketing *everything* as "healthy."

Look at VitaminWater as an example. These bottles contain a vast amount of vitamin B—great! But the issue is that this small assortment of vitamins does not justify VitaminWater's high sugar content—standing at 32.5 grams—included inside each bottle.

Our advice? Avoid them as much as you can. Get a water bottle instead. If you actually want added vitamins and minerals, take a supplement.

"Your breakfast is low in sugar": Flavored yogurt looks like the perfect breakfast or snack for a guy on the go—it combines fruits high in antioxidants with protein-packed dairy. However, flavored yogurt has a shockingly high sugar content. Flavored instant oatmeal has a similar issue. Some companies even proudly stamp their product cartons with the American Heart Association (AHA) checkmark. But if you look closely, you will find that what it *actually* complies with is the AHA's "food criteria for saturated fat and cholesterol."

So, your breakfast might have the same amount of sugar as Fruitloops do but still bears that AHA emblem with pride. The last thing you want to eat in your breakfast is sugar, a poor-quality refined carb that is going to raise your blood sugar levels and leave you hungry for more.

"Food containers are safe": Bisphenol (BPA), a synthetic chemical present in plastic and the lining of aluminum cans, is thought to be present in the bodies of 93 percent of Americans (The Healthy Journal, n.d.). Studies have confirmed BPA is linked to conditions including diabetes, obesity, mental problems, reduced sperm count, heart disease, and an elevated risk of breast, prostate, and testicular cancer, among other things.

According to recent research by the Environmental Working Group, BPA levels in one out of every ten food cans and one out of every three baby formula cans were more than two hundred times the government's recommended permitted exposure to industrial chemicals. (MacPherson, 2020). So, now what? The solution is simple. Purchase fresh or frozen vegetables and products stores in glass bottles or containers.

"Calorie counts are accurate": The FDA is more likely to sanction a food producer for overstating the net weight of a product than for underestimating it. Therefore, manufacturers tend to include more food than is indicated by the net weight on the package, or they make portions heavier than the serving size weight.

Try this yourself. Next time you return from the grocery shop, check the actual net weights and serving sizes of a few products on a standard food scale. You will probably find that a few of the items are heavier than they should be—meaning you're consuming more calories than you thought you were. We're not going to tell you to measure everything you buy but do keep this information in mind.

"Fruit juice is full of fruit": Do you still believe it when companies claim their juice is "100% pure"? While apple, grape, and pear juices are cheap, plentiful, and sugar-heavy, pomegranate, blueberry, and acai are more expensive and of greater quality, with lower sugar content. So, what do beverage companies do? They mix high-quality products with low-quality ones. Yes, it's still 100 percent pure and 100 percent juice, but it's actually a mixture of cheap, sugary juices that have been flavored lightly.

Only up to 20 percent of fruit drinks are actually made from real fruit juice; the remainder is sugar. Consider the hybrid juices offered by Ocean Spray; the majority contain close to 85 percent sugar. Rather than considering them as healthy fruit juices, you should just see them as non-carbonated soft drinks.

"All food additives are harmless" : According to researchers at the University of Southampton in the UK, artificial food coloring and the preservative sodium benzoate are directly linked to a rise in childhood hyperactivity (Food Standards Agency, n.d.).

In the US, packaged foods usually include the following additives:

- Yellow #5
- Yellow #6
- Red #40
- Sodium benzoate

Researchers are unsure whether a mixture of these chemicals or a single one is to blame for problems in children. You can find Red #40, Yellow #5, and Yellow #6 in Lucky Charms, while sodium benzoate can be found in pickles, jellies, and diet sodas.

"Artificial sweeteners are better for you": Don't want to eat sugar? Try artificial sweeteners; they're great for you. Not! Even though Diet Coke is essentially calorie-free, calorie-free beverages still contain certain properties and ingredients that can lead to weight gain. After analyzing the data gathered from 622 participants, researchers at the University of Texas Health Science Center discovered that consuming one can of diet soda per day resulted in a 41 percent increase in the likelihood of obesity (Fowler 2015).

Put simply, artificial sweeteners are not what you think they are. While they *are* better than normal sweets, there are better, healthier options out there.

The goal of this chapter was not to scare you about food and nutrition but to educate you. Your objective should now be to develop the mentality to eat healthier and wiser using the knowledge provided in this chapter. You can still eat whatever you want to but in a more informed and smarter manner.

CHAPTER 5

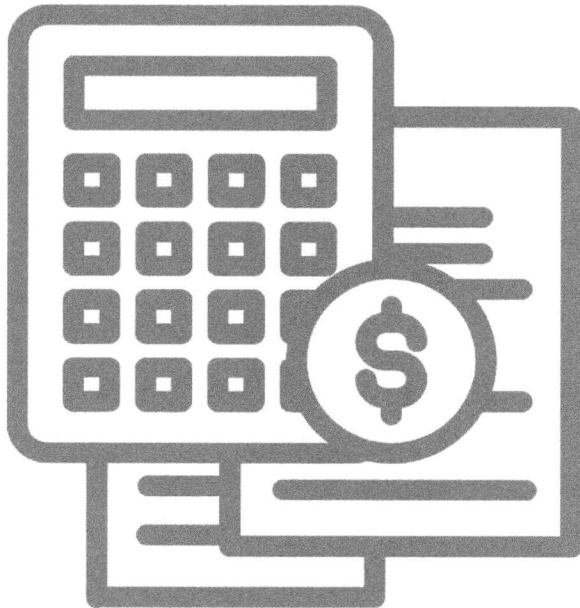

PERSONAL FINANCE

5

PERSONAL FINANCE

There is no room for Personal Finance 101 in our educational system—not in high schools or even in the best colleges or graduate programs. There are so many focused and talented men who fail to reach the pinnacle of success because of their lack of financial literacy. Financial education should be a crucial element of our education system, but it isn't.

There is so much biased and poor financial advice circling around the internet, so you cannot become properly educated just by watching YouTube videos. Financial advice all too often misses the larger picture and concentrates just on investing.

We are not here to offer you a get-rich-quick scheme. Instead, we want to help you connect your financial goals and challenges to your life goals since money is not an end in itself.

If you truly want to unleash the Beast Mode and live a healthy and sound life, you must have a thorough grasp of personal finance covering all aspects of your financial life, including spending, taxes, saving and investing, insurance, and making big financial plans for things like retirement, education, and home ownership. In this chapter, we discuss detailed, tried-and-true suggestions so that you can live a financially-free life no matter how much you earn.

EXPLORING THE ROOT CAUSES OF FINANCIAL IGNORANCE

Financial literacy is an important skill that impacts everyone, yet 57 percent of US adults struggle with low levels of financial knowledge. Since you are never going to be taught about money, you have to learn it for yourself. Don't be put off by thinking finance is too complex for you to understand. It isn't. Anybody who wants to learn about it can and should acquire financial literacy. Understanding finance can help you use your financial assets to your advantage and make wise financial decisions.

However, there are several reasons why many people lack financial knowledge. Many parents are not financially literate, and don't teach their children about money management. Some parents feel that money is an adult issue, and kids should not get involved. Additionally, some families don't talk about money at all, which can transmit ignorance, anxiety, and secrecy about the subject.

Unfortunately, the lack of financial education at home is not rectified by schools, as personal finance courses are not offered. This creates a cycle of financial ignorance that is passed down from generation to generation, and the education system is doing little to change it despite its practicality for real-life situations.

MONEY MASTERY IN MOTION

Bad money habits can not only be a source of great frustration and harm, but they stop you from realizing your dreams. However, bad money habits can be broken just like any other bad habit. First, you just need to recognize which of your behaviors are working against you.

Here are some tips on how to take your power back with your finances and some common bad habits men are typically guilty of:

Not sticking to a budget—or not having one in the first place.

Your monthly budget is your financial guide and will help you make better financial decisions. When you don't have a budget, you lack a solid grasp of your financial condition, making it much easier to fall into vicious spending habits. Budgeting helps you manage your money and ensure that your short- and long-term financial goals are met.

The solution is pretty simple. Set up a budget and make a commitment to stick to it. A common budgeting tactic is the 50/30/20 rule—this implies 50 percent of your budget goes to needs, 30 percent toward wants, and 20 percent toward savings. You won't need to check everything on an itemized basis each month if you keep the 30 and 20 percent separate from the 50 percent. When planning for this, it's also good practice to underestimate your monthly income a little to give you some wiggle room. Below is a simple exercise to get started with your budgeting.

Budgeting 101:

1. Run the numbers. Go through your bank and credit card statements and calculate your income. If you're paid on a regular basis, add up the previous month's paychecks; if your income is irregular, take your average for the last three to six months.
2. Establish short- and long-term financial objectives. It's important you know what you want to do with your money. Are you anxious to clear off your debt quickly? Are you considering buying a new house? Are you looking to make

room for more investments? Ask yourself questions to find out what your financial objectives are.

3. Keep an eye on your expenditures. This is important for both setting and following your budget. Choose a strategy to keep tabs on your expenditure, such as using a budgeting app or a spreadsheet. It's critical to gather all your income and spending data in one location to make it simpler to monitor. Also, make sure to schedule a time to review your budget at least once a month.

Having no emergency fund.

Emergencies hit us when we least expect them, and an emergency fund is a cash reserve put away for unforeseen events. Whether it's an unexpected medical expense, a broken appliance, a lost job, or even a sick cat, you never know when a financial emergency may arise and you need access to cash quickly to get you through a sticky situation. Even so, many educated and qualified individuals are reluctant to build an emergency fund.

It is estimated that more than 25 percent of Americans don't have a single dollar in their emergency fund (Egan 2020). What they don't realize is that having no emergency fund can put you in very challenging financial scenarios. For instance, it can force you to use a high-interest credit card to pay for a medical bill or mean you fall behind on your rent.

If you don't have an emergency fund, don't beat yourself up. Creating an emergency fund is simple. General rule of thumb is to work out 3-6 months of living expenses and have separate savings account, that you cannot easily access, with the equivalent amount of funds sitting in it to access during emergencies only.

Here is what you need to do:

1. Calculate your total monthly expenses.

2. Multiply it by six (for six months). If your monthly expenses are $1,500, aim for $9,000.
3. Start putting a part of your income into the emergency fund every month with the goal of building up to $9,000.

The difficult part of having an emergency fund is actually building it. Don't stress; start with what you can afford, and be sure to contribute on a regular basis. Work out what you can afford, and then set aside the money every week. When your budget allows for it, you can add more.

Spending more than you can afford.

You are not supposed to spend more than you can afford to. This seems so obvious, but so many people get this wrong. We are not advising you to be extremely frugal, but you need to understand what is and is not within your financial capabilities. According to a 2019 survey from Ladder, a life insurance company, people spend roughly eighteen thousand dollars annually on things that they don't need (Egan 2020). That's about fifty dollars a day.

Spending on non-essentials reduces the money available for paying necessities such as your mortgage or rent, credit card debt, school loans, and retirement. You should spend *some* money on your hobbies; in fact, it's a component of almost every healthy and happy existence. However, you need to make sure it doesn't get out of hand.

While it seems straightforward, life sometimes gets in the way. Here are some tips to help you on your way to having control over your finances.

Use cash: Purchasing with cash is more psychologically painful than paying with a credit card. That's why cash users tend to spend less than those who use cards. When you use a card, you don't necessarily feel anything since the process is so seamless, and there is no physical exchange. On the contrary, when you use cash, you literally see money being exchanged. This feeling of losing something prevents impulsive urges to buy more non-essential goods.

Pause before you buy: Every time you make a purchase, it is important you take a moment to think about it. Ask yourself the following questions:

- Is this a *need* or *want?*
- If it's a *want,* is it truly affordable?
- Would this purchase stop me from making deposits to my savings account?
- Would this result in me accruing additional credit card debt?

If any of the answers to these inquiries make you second guess your decision, consider delaying the purchase for now.

You also need to avoid giving in to discounts. Making savings is tempting; we get that. But it's important that you realize you don't save money by buying an item on sale unless you actually need it. You lose it.

Review your memberships and subscriptions: According to a Ladder poll, Americans spend more than $325 a month on memberships and subscriptions. This includes cable TV, online streaming platforms (ie. Netflix, Disney + etc), gym memberships and so on. Most people don't even use half of these subscriptions, so reducing them can result in annual savings of hundreds or even thousands of dollars that can be used toward more urgent requirements. Take thirty minutes from your day and work on this today! Cancel all subscriptions that you do not need.

Accumulating more and more debt.

According to Experian statistics, as of September 2022, the typical American had $96,371 in debt (Gillespie and Rubloff, 2023). It has now become part of American culture that you accumulate large debt and then strive to pay it off. These debts include credit card payments and personal and student loans. Financially illiterate men let these debts accumulate and pay off the minimum payment each month. Whether they realize it or not, they're paying more in interest over time.

Don't feel horrible if you have a mountain of debt on your shoulders. The Beast Mode mentality is not about feeling depressed; it is about acknowledging things are hard and still finding ways to make a change. Here are some ways you can take charge of your debts:

- **Eliminate debt:** Start by making a list of every loan you have, together with the yearly interest rate and the payment deadline for each. Now develop a strategy to make room in your budget to pay off those debts. You could choose to give more priority to those with higher interest or those with smaller balances.
- **Pay more than the required minimum:** Although making just the minimum payment due on your credit card bills each month may sound enticing, doing so will cost you a *ton* of interest. So, whenever you can, pay off your debt in full each month. By paying more than the minimum, you will reduce your interest costs and accelerate repayment.

Not saving for the future.

We have talked about saving for your emergency fund, but you also need to save for the future. At some point in your life, you might want to buy a house, get a car, or put your kids through college. You also don't want to work forever; you want to settle down and retire. Achieving these goals involves years of preparation and decades of saving.

Yet, most of America is not prepared for the future. According to a 2019 poll by Northwestern Mutual, 22 percent of Americans aged twenty-five and older have less than five thousand dollars saved for retirement, and 15 percent have no retirement savings at all (Egan, 2020). If you have no savings, you are certainly not alone. However, remember that not having a savings account may have the following consequences:

- Being unable to purchase a home
- Being unable to make a significant contribution to your children's college costs
- Having a delayed retirement or forced to remain in the workforce longer than desired

The good news is it's never too late to save for the future. You can start today. Here are some more tips to help you:

Automate your savings: You may be able to automatically transfer a portion of your income to a savings account that produces interest, depending on the function your bank provides. This makes the process hassle-free, and you don't have to worry about actively putting money in your savings account every month.

Trim your expenses: Look for ways to cut spending. For instance, stop paying for any unused subscriptions, look for the lower house and auto insurance, restructure your mortgage or auto loan, or consolidate your debt.

Get a side hustle: We don't want to put extra pressure on you. But if your financial state requires it, you could always consider getting a second job to complement your regular income and free up additional cash for savings. With the rise of remote work, taking on freelance gigs is an option.

Focus on your retirement funds: What can you do if you feel like you're falling behind on your retirement savings? If your employer offers a 401(k), take full advantage of it. Consider starting your own Individual Retirement Account (IRA) and contributing to it on a regular basis if a 401(k) is not an option for you; both are methods for long-term saving that will increase your contributions via investment. These funds will be available for withdrawal once you reach retirement age.

If you are trying to identify your bad financial practices, it implies that you are already making progress, regardless of the direction you go in. As there's no one-size-fits-all approach to managing money, you'll need to use some creativity and critical thinking skills to figure out how to get ahead financially. Two excellent places to start are by tracking your expenditure and credit.

WEALTH CONSCIOUSNESS UNLEASHED

Our whole lives, we are taught that money is scarce or something to be feared. Our beliefs about money shortages and our comparisons with others who may or may not have their own problems leads us to self-sabotage. Reframing your money mindset is not going to suddenly make you a millionaire, but it can help you handle the money you already earn more effectively. Learning to reframe how you think about money will help you feel more financially secure. Here are some toxic money thought patterns and how you can reframe them:

Reframe "spending" as "investing."

If you're like most Americans, you are always worried when you have to spend something. This is because people with little to no financial education tend to believe they are losing something they will never get back. When you bear that mindset, you develop a phobia of spending. In a lot of cases, *spending* is really *investing*. Therefore, whenever you spend any money, it is important to ask yourself:

- is it a wise investment? And,
- how much return will I get on my investment?

Your investment doesn't necessarily have to be in anything financial. You could choose to invest in yourself to boost your self-esteem and maintain your mental health. Think through all the ways you're spending money and all the returns you're getting. This way of thinking is also a fantastic way to spot expenses lacking any true return on investment so you can trim excessive spending such as unused subscriptions.

Change the language you use about money.

It's important we choose the language we use to discuss money carefully. You will often find yourself saying things such as:

"I can't afford it."

"I wish I had the money to go on a trip, but I don't."

"I can't afford to purchase those new clothes."

Since the expression "can't" derives from a position of scarcity, it has an impact on our actions and mentality as it implies inability.

Although there are certain things we absolutely cannot afford, we might theoretically afford the object or experience we're discussing by foregoing other expenses, utilizing savings, or borrowing money. Most of the time, we *choose* not to buy it. So instead of using the word "can't," we need to use the phrase we're "choosing not to." This is a far more powerful expression.

When you decide against doing something, you do it from a position of strength and abundance—a sign of a sound financial mindset. You've considered your alternatives and decided on the course of action that will offer you the most pleasure and happiness in the long run.

Develop an abundance mentality.

If you have a scarcity mindset, no amount of money can ever make you happy. You will always want to make more as there will always be more products and experiences you desire. We all love seeing our income rise. In fact, not only do we love it, but we tend to believe that increased income is the solution to all our problems. Think about it for a second. If your income tripled, you would finally be able to pay off your credit card debt, start saving significantly, or purchase the things you always wanted. However, this is a fantasy.

A study conducted at Vanderbilt University found that the bankruptcy rate among lottery winners is triple that of the general population. Within five years of winning, so many lottery winners find themselves back where they started or worse (Girlboss, n.d.). So what do you think went wrong for these lottery winners? They finally had the solution to all their problems, but they managed to blow it off. You are probably thinking they were a bunch of idiots but, in reality you would likely do the same.

When we have a scarcity mindset, we put boundaries all around us. We keep telling ourselves no until we finally rebel and lose control. This means we make impulsive purchases that trap us in a loop of feeling terrible and restricting ourselves again and prevent us from meeting our financial goals.

To stop this pattern, we need to shift to an abundance mentality. It's a subtle change, but it will help you stop desiring and demanding the stuff you've always wanted. Bearing an abundance mindset, the serial shopper loses the desire to shop, and the so-called coffee junkie skips the fancy store-bought coffee. But why is the abundance mentality so powerful?

When we reframe our mindset and believe that we already have more than enough, we become conscious of the wealth we already possess. It's an eye-opening exercise that will make you feel so much better about yourself and your financial condition.

Stop with the comparison.

We have addressed comparison throughout this book, but it's worth repeating. It's so easy to fall prey to comparison in this era of social media, reality TV, and celebrity publications. We constantly make comparisons between ourselves and other members of our family, our acquaintances, famous people, and TV characters.

When you compare your wealth with someone else's, you compare what you know about yourself (i.e., everything) with what you *see* of someone else (i.e., the side they choose to show on social media). You can only predict that someone is living the high life based on their social media posts and can't ever really know their financial situation. Someone may seem to have a wonderful life full of expensive clothing, trips, and other enjoyable things on the surface, but their lifestyle may really be powered by credit card debt or worse! Not everything that glitters is gold.

Comparing yourself with others will also cultivate a scarcity mindset and means you lose sight of your own goals. Instead, it's likely you'll fall into the trap of trying to "look rich" instead of working to achieve wealth. It is important to realize that everyone has their own timeline. Your friend might have bought his own house at twenty, while you have to wait till you are forty-five. There is no shame in that.

Create realistic objectives for yourself and measure your progress against only yourself. Enjoy your achievements along the way and revise your financial goals as you progress.

The budget mentality.

From what we've seen throughout the years, there are two types of budgeters:

1. People with no budget. Even when they do create one, they are unable to follow it and give in to frivolous spending without any second thoughts.
2. People so strict about their budget that it leave no room for fun.

You don't have to be either of these. The first type of people are losing their key to financial freedom, and the latter are losing their chance to be happy.

The goal of a budget is to help you learn about your finances and to guide your spending so you can save for the future without falling into debt. Yes, the budget needs to have boundaries, but the boundaries need to be optimized to allow for happiness. After all, the end goal of money is to give you financial freedom.

Ironically, boundaries will liberate you because knowing where your money is and goes gives you far more control over your finances. If going out to dinner once a week makes you happy, allocate money in your budget to cover the expense. You can adjust your spending to make sure you're allocating your hard-earned money to the things that matter most to you. We sometimes spend money on things that don't genuinely make us happy, even though we think they will. This is why we need to be clear on how much of our budget we use on ourselves and whether the object or experience actually makes us happy or not.

BEAST MODE MENTALITY TO CONQUERING YOUR FINANCES

We have nearly covered everything you need to do to be at the top of your finances. We talked about creating a budget, sticking to a budget, and paying off debt, among other things. But the point of this book is to guide you toward taking action, so here is an action plan for you to follow so that you never lag behind in your finances anymore:

Be paid what you are worth.

You want to get paid as much as you can, and that's all right; we all want that. Start by demanding enough to cover a fair standard of living. This may vary depending on where you choose to live, but "decent" typically means having enough money to cover your mortgage or rent, investing in a family, being able to fill up a vehicle with gas, and eating whatever you want whenever you want. And to state the obvious, being able to save at least 20 percent of your income in addition to your emergency fund. It is important to note that once you achieve this standard of living, having more money will not make you any happier, but earning less will make you unhappy.

Nobody will understand your worth more than you. Ask yourself: are you worth more or less than you're currently being paid? In the case you are underearning, you are losing money every single day. You can access information on wages on websites like Salary.com and Monster.com. We recommend asking someone in a rival company how much people are earning their company for the same position you're in.

Now you know what you're worth, it's time for job hunting. Job hunting is an important aspect of your financial condition. The first thing to do is to take advantage of every chance that sounds worthwhile. Researchers from Columbia University and Swarthmore College interviewed students graduating from college who were looking for employment and discovered that those who pursued perfection often received positions earning 20 percent more than their counterparts. This makes sense because the more clarity you have regarding the job you want, the more likely you are to land a role paying you what you're worth. The less choosy you are about your job, the more likely it is that your position will fall short of expectation.

If you have been in your job for a few years, there's a high chance you are now underpaid. If this is the case, consider "upskilling". This involves learning new skills that can complement your existing role and makes you more of an asset for the company that you work for. You will sure to be noticed with the higher ups when you are doing more than the minimum and offering more value than your colleagues and have a higher chance at a raise or a promotion.

Save on a schedule.

Think about it for a second. There is so much to do in life. Buy a home, get married, have children, bring them up, pay for their education, have fun, and travel the world. When you think about all the things you need to do, you will understand that life is expensive. But it's not unaffordable if you are smart about it.

First things first: when you get your paycheck, put 20 percent of it into your savings accounts immediately. Do this before paying your bills or withdrawing any money. If you cannot manage to save 20 percent, at least make a habit of saving 10 to 15 percent. As your savings account grows, you will be more encouraged to save.

This habit of saving becomes much easier when you know what you are saving for. Earning money stimulates the reward centers in your brain, but saving for the future does not. It's no wonder people are so terrible at it. So, when you are saving money for a purpose, you can visualize the outcome and stimulate the reward center . Remember, it doesn't matter how small your goals are. Overly ambitious goals are a key factor in why so many people struggle to save money.

When it comes to savings, you should stop focusing on things you can't control. Stop focusing on the stock market or the interest rates. Focus on the things you *can* control, such as the year you start saving or the quantity you save. Why? Suppose you start making monthly investments of $250 at the age of twenty-five and earn an imaginary 6 percent interest. You'll have saved approximately $340,000 by the time you're sixty. Let's imagine you delay until age thirty-five and increase your savings by 20 percent ($300 per month), and the interest rate gets increased to 9 percent. By the time you are sixty, guess how much money you will have? $308,000. The takeaway: the sooner you start saving, the longer you will have the power of compounding interest working in your favor. This means you will save more money in the long term.

Be careful of debts.

The idea is simple—don't spend more than you make. Debt puts you in a vicious cycle, which is *exactly* where credit card companies want you to be. While there are definitely good debts and bad debts, the rule to remember is that every debt is costly. Yes, even the ones with 0 percent interest. When you take a loan, you are pledging a portion of your future earnings. What else might you have done with the $379 a month you spend on the second card? Over a month, nothing much, but over sixty months? How much money would that have accumulated to be had you saved it and leveraged off the compounding interest?

Although we say debt is always bad, there are still times when it's unavoidable, and you need a loan. Good debts are those which put a certificate on your wall, wheels under your feet, or a roof over your head. But being in debt for buying a new refrigerator when you already have two definitely does not fall under the definition of good debt. Poor debt management is the reason so many people fail to succeed financially even when they are earning six figures.

How responsible you are with your debts is represented by your credit score. Keeping a good credit score will help you save so much money in the long run. A good credit score is easier to build than you think. Here is what you need to do to protect your credit score and qualify for better interest rates:

- Pay your payments on time.
- Stop using more than 30 percent of your credit limit.
- Don't open additional cards just for the sake of it.
- Keep cards open even if you aren't using them.

Sound simple? It is.

Start investing.

Congratulations! You have done everything right. You made a budget, cleared your debts, and are saving enough. Now what? Well, now it's time for your money to help you make *more* money.

When we pitch the idea of investing, most men are afraid because they have never done it before. People only believe what they hear in the media, and the media only talks about how the whole global economy is going down. So, it is pretty common to feel frightened about investing. And even if you are convinced and don't already invest, you probably have no idea where to start.

First things first: keep your investing game as simple as possible. Don't try to be smart with it; just focus on creating a boring portfolio. We are pretty sure you've heard about index funds and ETFs. These index funds and ETFs closely follow a collection of equities that are related to one another, such as the S&P 500. They move up and down slowly. Nonetheless, these funds are inexpensive to hold, trade, and tax. Historically, simply investing in an index fund like S&P 500 has always worked out better than picking out individual stocks. You don't have to have good instincts and extensive market knowledge. Invest a small portion of your income into the S&P 500 each month and see your money grow in the long term.

There is a chance that you will run out of money during your retirement. Reduce your chances by automating your investment contributions and raising your percentages when your income rises. If you've never saved before and money is tight, start with 3 percent and then raise it by 2 percent each year until you reach your maximum commitment of 15 percent. If you're over forty and haven't yet begun investing, it's time to clench your teeth and start super saving. Your odds of running out of money decrease to 20 percent after only twenty years of 401(k) contributions ("Men's health," 2011).

Many of us believe that financial freedom is about earning more money. And yes, earning more money does help, but it is more about the way you *manage* that money. Your financial attitudes and habits are key indicators of whether you will be able to fulfill your financial goals. Learning to manage your finances is important for every man, and by using the Beast Mode mindset explored in this chapter, you will be well on your way to financial stability, which will serve as a foundation for the rest of your aspirations.

CONCLUSION

You must have a strong mentality able to continue when faced with adversity, a healthy body that is fit and well-fed, and a solid grasp on your personal finances to liberate you and allow you to achieve greatness. We have debunked some of the most widespread stereotypes about men, including those claiming that men are emotionless, uncaring, and domineering. We have also explored aspects of the modern man's lifestyle, including physical fitness, health and nutrition, and personal finance.

This book provides the essential tools to overcome your challenges in these areas and develop grit, passion, and determination. Results won't happen overnight, but if you utilize the knowledge contained in this book and really work to improve yourself, you'll get to where you need to be.

Beast Mode is a mentality. It is the ultimate attitude to help men overcome limiting beliefs and encourage personal growth. Men face immense pressures today to excel professionally while maintaining fulfilling personal relationships. They are also placed under stress to be resilient, self-assured, and strong, as well as perceptive, compassionate, and emotionally responsive. Finding this balance can be incredibly difficult, but we sincerely hope that reading the first book in our *Beast Mode for the Modern Man* series has given you tools to deal with the worry, tension, and anxiety caused by the demands of daily life.

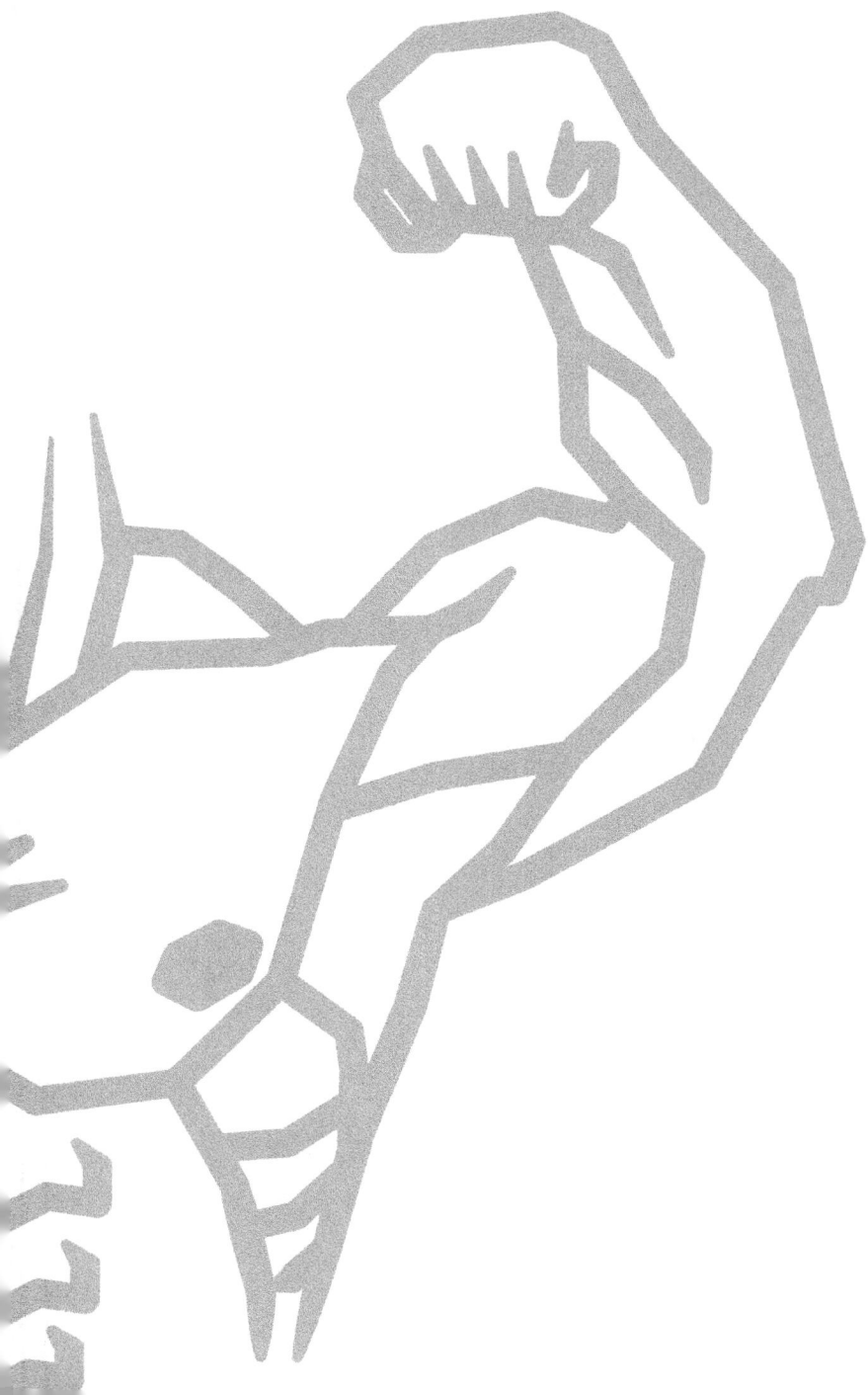

REFERENCES

"Actions of caffeine in the brain with special reference to factors that contribute to its widespread use." n.d. PubMed. Accessed February 19, 2023. https://pubmed.ncbi.nlm.nih.gov/10049999/.

Anderson, MW. n.d. "Alleviation of sleep maintenance insomnia with timed exposure to bright light." PubMed. Accessed February 19, 2023. https://pubmed.ncbi.nlm.nih.gov/8340561/.

"Anxiety Disorders - Facts & Statistics." n.d. Anxiety and Depression Association of America. Accessed February 18, 2023. https://adaa.org/about-adaa/press-room/facts-statistics.

Butler, Kelsey. 2018. "7 Effects of Sleep Deprivation - What No Sleep Does to Your Body." Men's Health. https://www.menshealth.com/health/g23414448/effects-of-sleep-deprivation/.

Egan, John. 2020. "5 Bad Money Habits and How to Break Them." Experian. https://www.experian.com/blogs/ask-experian/bad-money-habits-and-how-to-break-them/.

Food Standards Agency. n.d. "Food additives." Food Standards Agency. Accessed March 9, 2023. https://www.food.gov.uk/safety-hygiene/food-additives#food-colours-and-hyperactivity.

Fowler, Sharon P. 2015. "Diet soda intake is associated with long-term increases in waist circumference in a bi-ethnic cohort of older adults: The San Antonio Longitudinal Study of Aging." NCBI. https://www.ncbi.nlm.nih.gov/pmc/articles/PMC4498394/.

Gillespie, Lane, and Tori Rubloff. 2023. "Average American Debt Statistics." Bankrate. https://www.bankrate.com/personal-finance/debt/average-american-debt/.

Girlboss. n.d. "Want To Reframe Your Money Mindset Once And For All? Start Here." Girlboss. Accessed March 10, 2023. https://girlboss.com/blogs/read/reframe-your-money-mindset.

"Goal setting as a strategy for dietary and physical activity behavior change: a review of the literature." n.d. PubMed. Accessed February 27, 2023. https://www.ncbi.nlm.nih.gov/pubmed/15559708.

Gough, Brendan. 2006. "'Real men don't diet': An analysis of contemporary newspaper representations of men, food and health." sciencedirect.com. https://www.sciencedirect.com/science/article/abs/pii/S0277953606004795.

"Gym workouts for beginners." 2019. Nuffield Health. https://www.nuffieldhealth.com/article/gym-workouts-for-beginners#beginner-gym-workout-for-strength.

The Healthy Journal. n.d. "What percentage of Americans have BPA in their bodies?" The Healthy Journal. Accessed March 9, 2023. https://www.thehealthyjournal.com/faq/what-percentage-of-americans-have-bpa-in-their-bodies.

Johnson, Dagny. n.d. "Caffeine maintains vigilance and improves run times during night operations for Special Forces." PubMed. Accessed February 19, 2023. https://pubmed.ncbi.nlm.nih.gov/16018347/.

Legg, Timothy J., and Raj Dasgupta. 2018. "4-7-8 Breathing: How It Works, How to Do It, and More." Healthline. https://www.healthline.com/health/4-7-8-breathing#How-to-do-it-.

Loveific. n.d. "Home." YouTube. Accessed March 11, 2023. https://www.loveific.com/guys-only-want-one-thing/.

MacPherson, Rachel. 2020. "What Is BPA? the Dangerous Chemical Found in 10% of Canned Foods." Insider. https://www.insider.com/guides/health/diet-nutrition/what-is-bpa.

Majaski, Christian. 2019. "Study: Men Are Overworking Themselves to Death." askmen.com. https://www.askmen.com/news/health/study-men-are-overworking-themselves-to-death.html.

McClain, Maurice. 2019. "What does anxiety look like in men?" Edward-Elmhurst Health. https://www.eehealth.org/blog/2019/09/men-anxiety/.

"Money Management Tips for Men." 2011. Men's Health. https://www.menshealth.com/trending-news/a19517584/money-management-tips/.

Morse, Anne M., Kate Robards, and Katherine Robards. 2023. "Does sleep deprivation make you more manly?" Sleep Education. https://sleepeducation.org/does-sleep-deprivation-make-you-more-manly/.

Nelson, Audrey. 2022. "Failure and Burnout Are Tough on Men." Psychology Today. https://www.psychologytoday.com/us/blog/he-speaks-she-speaks/202205/failure-and-burnout-are-tough-on-men.

Oettingen, Gabrielle. 2009. "Mental Contrasting and Goal Commitment: The Mediating Role of Energization." *Sage Journals* 35, no. 5 (February). https://doi.org/10.1177/0146167208330856.

"One in 100 deaths is by suicide." 2021. World Health Organization (WHO). https://www.who.int/news/item/17-06-2021-one-in-100-deaths-is-by-suicide.

"President's Council on Sports, Fitness & Nutrition." n.d. Office of Disease Prevention and Health Promotion. Accessed February 26, 2023. https://health.gov/our-work/nutrition-physical-activity/presidents-council.

Robards, Kate, and David Troy. 2023. "How sleep disorders affect men's health." Sleep Education. https://sleepeducation.org/how-sleep-disorders-affect-mens-health/.

Sayer, Amber. 2022. "These are the best workouts for beginners so you can build a solid routine." The Manual. https://www.themanual.com/fitness/best-workouts-for-beginners/.

"10 Worst Diet Excuses | realbuzz.com." n.d. Realbuzz. Accessed March 3, 2023. https://www.realbuzz.com/articles-interests/nutrition/article/10-worst-diet-excuses/.

Weber, Joel, Mike Zimmerman, and Editors of Men's Health Magazi. 2010. *The Men's Health Big Book of Food & Nutrition: Your Completely Delicious Guide to Eating Well, Looking Great, and Staying Lean for Life!* N.p.: Harmony/Rodale.